Breast Cancer
and Me

a product of learning to give and take. It did not happen overnight.

God took a country girl and a city boy with totally different heritages and melted them into one. The crucible was typical, everyday family life: starving through college, forming career paths, raising three boys, volunteering in community service and learning to walk faithfully with our Lord. We trusted God continually to perfect the work He had begun in each of us.

We always felt a good relationship was worth fighting for. Many times the "fighting for" took hours. Behind our closed bedroom door. Accusations, hurt feelings, disparity over child rearing or remorse over the budget. We fought, emptying our gunnysacks of grievances, with each other periodically over thirty-four years. God brought us through.

Now our relationship is worn comfortably—like old tennis shoes. We have learned to nourish and care for "us" as we would a priceless heirloom. We consider spending time together a blessing from God.

When our last child left home, I wrote about the experience in my weekly newspaper column:

> We have entered a new era in our home. We are alone. ALONE TO-GETHER. Just him and me and the two cats and twenty-six ducks.
>
> Our sons are officially raised. I think. At least they are no longer here for meals.

The youngest started college this fall. He now has his own pad.

The middle son graduated from college in June. He spent two months at home while seeking a job. That two months endangered our mother-son relationship at many times, but we did survive. Now he has a job and a pad too.

This first night of ALONE TOGETHER should have been a special occasion. We had looked forward to this for twenty-six years. No, that is not true.

We didn't start looking forward to being alone until we had teenagers. But with each progressing year, ALONE TOGETHER kept looking better.

Right now, let me state that we dearly love our children—and almost all of the time. But I think the idea is to raise them up and then they leave. Then the father and mother can spend some time together with the love they share that started this whole thing to begin with!

I knew I should cook something special and have candles and a tablecloth and all . . . but I was just exhausted. The summer had not been easy. I reheated some leftover hot dogs. Robert said he didn't mind. He was exhausted too. After supper he stretched out on the couch. I curled up on the love seat.

Our first night ALONE TOGETHER af-

ter all these years. He slept. I slept. Finally
we got up and went to bed and slept. You
have heard of jet-lag? We must have had
parenting-lag.

"Time Out with Lois," reprinted from the *Rosebud
Press* and the *Forsyth Independent*, September 29,
1988.

The restaurant we chose for lunch was both
sophisticated and charming. One of the de-
lights of a day off together in Billings was picking a new place to dine. Between courses our
chatter was mostly about the new tape deck for
our car.

"You'd think we were teenagers," I said.
"Paying that much just so we could listen to all
our tapes."

"Nope," Robert said. "A teenager would have
spent twice that much!"

"You know another thing we should talk
about," I said between bites of savory crab
salad. "We could be facing cancer, you know."

"I don't think we should think that. Let's just
wait and see what Dr. Fina has to say."

"Well, I just feel like we should pray. Let's
ask God to have His perfect will in whatever
happens with the tests."

So we prayed a simple prayer, like so many
we had prayed together over the years. "Lord,
here we are. You know our future. Take care of
Lois. Give the doctors wisdom as they look at
the tests. In Your name, amen."

We picked up our car with our teenage tape deck and drove to the Billings clinic. When we walked into Dr. Fina's office, he had films up on the white screen in the exam room. His expression and manner immediately told us he didn't like what he was seeing. I thought he was upset.

"First, I want to take another look at you." He didn't look at my ears or my toes. He began another breast exam at once. The left breast. "Did you feel anything here?" he asked.

"No."

"Can you feel this?" He directed my hand to the top of my breast.

"Yes, I feel that. It feels like a mint. It's not round. It's flat and movable."

He went to the screen, again staring at the black and white film. His manner was entirely different from our usual comfortable bantering back and forth.

"I didn't feel it either this morning. But we obviously have a lump."

"We" must include me. I glanced at Robert. He looked pale green. "Are you OK?" I asked.

He just gave me a weak smile with, "Are *you* OK?" A little question with thirty years of togetherness in three words. Love. Concern. Grief. His "Are you OK?" was trembling.

"I have to tell you that some other doctors have looked at this," Dr. Fina said, "and we agree that it appears to be a malignant tumor."

"Can you see it on last year's film?" I questioned. "How old is this thing?"

"Tumors can grow for years before we can detect them," he said. He looked as pale as Robert. "There is not a sign of this on your mammogram which was in March last year. I checked." Dr. Fina put his hand on my shoulder. "Are you OK?"

"Yes," I said. "Yes, I'm fine. Well, I mean, I thought I was fine."

I tried to feel what I was feeling. (Can you understand that?) I didn't feel afraid. I didn't feel panic. I didn't feel doom hanging over my head. I just felt . . . I just felt . . . I just felt fine.

Dr. Fina was decidedly uncomfortable. I wanted to pat his shoulder and tell him it was OK. Did he feel bad because he had not felt the lump in the morning? Did he feel bad because he had told me how "healthy" I was just a few hours earlier? We didn't have time to talk.

He said, "I'll get the nurse. I have already called a surgeon. I want you to talk to him today."

The nurse had a sadder face than the doctor. She walked us down the hall and around the corner. Robert reached for my hand as we followed the nurse. We walked through the doorway that read Oncology Surgery Hematology.

Isn't this interesting (and that is the exact word that came to my mind), I thought as I followed the nurse, *I wonder what God has in mind now?* Inside there was a feeling of His presence surrounding me. It gave me such peace and a sense of security.

The nurse showed us to chairs in the waiting room. "Dr. Brown will be with you shortly," she said apologetically. She did not look reassuring as she walked away.

"Are you OK?" Robert asked, holding my hand tightly.

"I'm OK. Are you OK?"

"I am just worried about you," he said.

There was that "OK" question again. Multitudes of unanswerable questions in one.

"Well, if you want to know what I'm feeling right now, the truth is . . . I'm just thinking that God has opened a door into another room in my life." My eyes locked with his. "And I'm glad it's my door. Not your door. Or the door of one of our kids or their wives. Or my folks. It is me."

It will always be my belief that when serious illness attacks one in a couple, it is harder to be the spouse than the ill one. I knew what I was feeling. He had to wonder and imagine.

"Let's pray," I said.

There were four other people in our end of the waiting room. Three were engrossed in magazines. One man was sleeping. His head was slipping closer toward his chest as we sat there.

"Lord, we pray You will give us strength for what is ahead. We thank You that You are with us right now. We know You will walk with us in all that is in the future. In Jesus' name, amen."

The nurse came out. "It will be awhile yet before we can work you in," she apologized.

"That's OK, we're not going anywhere," Robert replied.

So we sat in the waiting room.

Waiting.

My mind was envisioning the future . . .

> *With cancer.*
> *My job.*
> *Robert.*
> *His job.*
> *Speaking engagements already booked—*
> *   two of them in less than ten days.*
> *The kids.*
> *My folks.*
> *Carol.*
> *Phyllis.*
> *Robert.*
> *Mary.*
> *Broom.*
> *Marilyn.*
> *Sharon.*
> *My church family.*
> *My boss.*
> *Robert.*

Oh Lord, this is going to affect a lot of people. Please help them walk this path also. Oh, please comfort Robert. Give him strength right now.

One by one the people were beckoned by the nurse to go around the corner and down the hall to the little rooms. I recalled the last time I was in this area of the clinic. I had brought my friend Kitty Berube for one of her chemotherapy treatments. She had later died from cancer. . . . That recollection started my mind down a path . . .

There is John Williams. . . .
    He had bone cancer. He is doing great. . . .

But there was my friend Pat Hofeldt. . . .
    She died from breast cancer. . . .

Connie Bailey had breast cancer. . . .
    She is doing good. Debbie is doing
good . . . and so is Fay . . .

        and so was *Kitty . . . and so* was *Pat .*

Bruce is hanging in there, and so is Cheryl
    Booth.

I looked over at Robert beside me. I wondered if his mind was reciting a cancer roll call too.

R-r-in-g-g, R-i-i-ng. "Hello, this is the Cancer Recruiter. I'm just calling to tell you that your number has been selected. . . ."

"Do you want to just go home tonight?" Robert asked, breaking the silence.

We had made reservations to stay two nights

in Billings. It was all written down in my notebook with two hearts drawn on the weekend.

---

*"Excuse me, did you get cancer penciled
in there?"*

"No. I want to stay," I told Robert. I don't
give my schedules up easily. "Besides I think
I'll need the ladies retreat tomorrow more than
ever. God will uplift me there."

"Mrs. Olmstead?"

We hopped up. We were the last ones in the
waiting room. It was nearly 5 o'clock. We had
sat there an hour and fifteen minutes. Thinking. Grasping each other's hand from time to
time. Waiting. There was a smile on my face, I
am sure, as I followed the nurse. I knew beyond a shadow of a doubt that God was in control. My Aunt Ruth had penned in her Bible,
"The will of God does not take us where the
grace of God cannot keep us."

So God was in control.

Right under God was this Dr. Brown.

We went into the little room to practice waiting some more. Waiting now for *the surgeon*. I
had never had surgery in my life. I had never
even had stitches. I wondered what this surgeon would be like. Images floated through my
mind . . . with face masks, sterile doctor-suits,
scalpels, (no, cancel that picture) . . . and the
face of Winchester from *M*A*S*H*. . . .

This definitely was going to be a new chapter in my life.

"I just do not understand it." Under the nurse's directive, I was taking my blouse off for the seventh time of the day.

"Do not understand what?" Robert was still looking serious.

"I cannot understand why, if they want to look at your front, they tell you to tie the gown in the back. Why can't you just put it on with the opening in the front?"

Finally there was the sound of paper rustling outside the door. A young man, with a smile and friendly eyes, wearing a white coat said, "I am Dr. Brown. I have one more patient to see. Then I can spend as long as we need, talking, OK?"

He shut the door. He didn't have a face mask on. No scalpel in his hand either.

"Yup. That's OK. I think *my* schedule is going down the drain," I said to the closed door.

We sat, staring at the wall, the cotton swabs, the packets of antiseptic cleanser, the sink, the wallpaper . . . and each other. Robert was starting to look normal again.

I shivered. The paper gown didn't provide much warmth. It was tied in the back too. I always follow directions when I'm intimidated. *Lord, this certainly is interesting. . . . I just have to smile, thinking about how You are going to use this for Your glory. Dear Father, You know how I am. You are going to have to do a mighty miracle within me. Let me be found faithful. . . .*

"Well, I think I'm about ready," I said to Robert. "I think I've about waited to the end of my capabilities. How about you?"

He picked a *Popular Science* magazine out of the rack. He had already gone through the three magazines in the rack a dozen times. His hands were shaking. "I think, let's get this show on the road."

"See, we told you tickets were available. Just look. You got front row seats!"

Chapter 2

Confronting Cancer

How do you feel when you hear your chart being pulled and the papers rustling outside your exam room door? Does your adrenalin race?

It might have been tough making that appointment. While in the waiting room, you feel less sick. Maybe you ought to tell them you'll just go home, see how you feel tomorrow. But just as you're about to sneak out, your name is called. You get escorted to that little exam room. You forget about leaving. Now you want to see the doctor and get your problem fixed . . . absolutely no different than going to the auto collision repair shop with your car.

"Here's the car. I'll be back tomorrow at four."

Only this body shop is different. There are no estimates or prices displayed in red or black on the wall. There are no catalogs to pick out the parts you need. You don't have to stay out of the shop area either. They tell you to come right in.

First, you get to see the nurse. The nurse gets your temperature and blood pressure. And you have to talk about the problem you really wanted to tell only to the doctor. The nurse grants you the privilege of wearing one of those designer gowns.

There is no question of running now. You go to bed at night dressed more decently than this! There is nothing to do but keep your ear tuned toward that chart box outside the door.

Then the door opens. The doctor is here.

*   *   *

He was definitely not Charles Emerson Winchester III. Alan Alda, maybe, with glasses. He shook Robert's hand as he passed through to the doctor-chair by the desk with the cotton swabs and tongue depressors. This surgeon was clad in the body of a regular person.

With just a few remarks and questions, first impressions registered on my mental chart: comfortable, friendly, unintimidating, professional . . . without a scalpel and face mask. *Thank You, Lord. Good work so far.*

Now let's see about the subject at hand. Cancer.

Dr. Brown apologized for the delay. "But now I am here. We can take as long as you want to go over all your options."

Two more points on the register, I think. *This is*

Friday night. He doesn't mind how long this takes? I might really like this doctor-surgeon-person.

For the next hour he explained our options. It was the first time the national statistics got personal. "One in nine women in America gets breast cancer now," he said. (As of 1996, that figure is one in eight women.)

"See, I told you we had lots of tickets. We're running a high-tech production here. Now listen what our casting director has in mind for you. . . ."

He carefully went over my lump, first physically examining it. He gave the various possibilities for treatment if it was malignant. Then we listened intently as he discussed the probabilities of the future. Now and then one of us broke in with a question.

It was different than viewing one of the American Cancer Society videos. It was different than listening to one of their advertisements on television. I was co-chairman of the Colstrip chapter of the American Cancer Society. I knew some cancer facts. I had read the brochures which I received after donating to their annual drive.

But this was different. This was me. My body.

Both Robert and I paid close attention. As a matter of fact, we were riveted on every word of Dr. Brown.

"I would say more than likely, from my experience, your lump is malignant. We will schedule a biopsy. This biopsy will be analyzed at the lab. You have choices. *If* it is malignant, you can have a lumpectomy, which is the removal of the lump and some of the surrounding tissue. Or you can have the entire breast removed which is called a mastectomy."

I was reassured since he spoke confidently and looked me in the eye.

"You don't have to decide right away. A week or two isn't going to make any difference. And let me just reiterate: There is no significant difference in the survival outcome of a mastectomy or a lumpectomy with adjuvant treatment. The statistics are basically the same."

I didn't think to ask what "adjuvant treatment" was.

With that he paused. "So this is up to you. What questions do you have?"

He had looked and talked to Robert as much as me. I was thankful for that. This was pretty serious stuff. He had pointed out to us the signs of probable malignancy on my mammogram.

"We won't be sure until we do the actual biopsy. And that's another option you have. After the biopsy you can wait a week or two to decide what you want to do. That could involve two operations, but it's up to you."

We listened to his observations and descriptions of treatment as if my life depended on it. *Weird, I guess it does!*

It was getting late. "Well, I'll tell you what, Dr. Brown," I said. "When I go to the beauty shop I tell them to do my hair however they think best. They're the professionals. I figure they know more than I do so I let them make the decision. That's how I feel about this. You tell us what you think is best."

He shook his head and tossed the ball right back in my court. "I won't do that. It's your body. It's your decision."

I looked at Robert. "What do you think?"

"What do *you* think?" he countered.

"I think the scale leans toward the lumpectomy."

"That's what I think," Robert said.

"Then let's just do it."

I turned to Dr. Brown to tell him our decision. He had already turned into Doctor-surgeon-answer-person-friend Brown.

"I imagine that you have plans for Saturday. So do I. Then I want to go to church on Sunday and have the elders anoint me with oil and pray for me, like it says in the Bible. . . . So how about Monday?"

He smiled. "The desk is closed now." It was well past 6. "But let's have you come in Monday at 9. I will see what we can do."

He looked at Robert. He looked at me. "You are sure? You don't want any more time to think about this?"

I was sure. I looked at Robert. He was looking at me. I could just feel his vibes of love
and empathy and concern. "You are sure?" I
asked.

"Let's do it," he said.

I loved him for the "let's" part.

I also knew God was with us so surely that I
could feel His presence in the little room. I was
ready to get alone with Him. We needed to
talk. We had some priorities to rearrange.

"Then we'll see you Monday," I said in fare-
well, for now, to this Dr. Brown-surgeon-per-
son. "I'll be praying for you . . . and me too."

And that was the real beginning. The wheels
were in motion. I could see one thing right
away. My notebook was definitely due for a rewrite. It looked like cancer wanted to be in my
schedule.

I wondered just how many pages it would
take?

Confronting Cancer—Application

It is the American way to try to assemble the
bookcase or the bicycle or the new tent first. If
that doesn't work, we look for the directions.
Last, we ask for help.

1. *Pray first.*

2. Ask questions. Don't rush your decision.

3. Be certain of your direction. God will give
   you peace about the right direction for you.

4. Be comfortable and confident about your doctor and your plan of attack.

5. Read every brochure and each piece of information the doctors give you.

6. Write down your questions for your doctors whenever you think of them. Otherwise you may forget.

I like to write down my feelings and thoughts. Then I review my notes as I pray. (See more on this subject in Chapter 13.) Use your Bible as a reference tool.

Bible References

Isaiah 41:13	Psalm 28:1, 7
Psalm 27	Romans 8:15
Romans 8:37-39	Psalm 23
Proverbs 29:25	John 14:27
Psalm 118:29	

I use the King James Version. Use the Bible translation with which you are most comfortable.

Chapter 3

The Weather Forecast and an Angel

We walked from the clinic back to the motel. The three of us. Robert, me and our uninvited guest. Cancer.

"You'll get used to me. I will not let you forget that I'm with you—you just may not know where. It's part of my job."

The unseasonably warm day spoke of spring and new life. Dusk was preparing to clothe us for another evening.

My life was changing even as we walked the short distance to the motel. The spring day in my own heart had a new forecast. A storm loomed ahead. We had just been through the weather update.

In Montana, we have a stockmen's advisory broadcast on radio and television when a severe storm is approaching. I suppose it would be similar to a tornado watch in other states. Whatever the name, I could hear the news.

I could feel the wind picking up, the air getting cooler, the sky darkening. I could see the clouds as they peeked over the horizon:

cancer

discomfort   distress   pain
tears   hurt   suffering
testing   sorrow
despair

Daylight was turning into dusk. But not just for me. This storm was going to cast its shadows on my friends and family. There was a new pain in my heart, thinking of having to tell them "the forecast."

It was the same blue and mauve motel room we had stayed in the night before. But it seemed different now. Robert turned on the brass and wood lamp. I sat down on the bed. It felt like a corporate board room.

He mixed a glass of iced tea for himself and poured a cup of coffee for me from our thermos. "Now what?" he asked as he sat down in the recliner at the end of the bed.

"Let's make the calls and then I want the special evening we had planned. . . . I *need* the evening we'd planned. Is that OK with you?"

I called my friend Carol first. She had moved from Kentucky to live and work in our community. We have different lifestyles. She is single. I am an old-married. She likes motorcycles, sports cars and outdoor sports. I like shopping, decorating, Victorian lace and flowers.

She has a demanding career as a physicians' assistant. For months she was our sole health care provider in a community of 3,300. My job is being a friendly receptionist, nothing like making health care decisions and fighting for a patient's life. My most extreme crisis at work is handling an irate customer who thought his street should have been plowed yesterday. Or it was plowed yesterday and now he has a huge pile of snow blocking his driveway!

Carol has an intense love for the Lord Jesus Christ. So do I. She hates to cook. So do I. She loves Bible study and prayer. So do I. And right now I needed a prayer.

"Hello?"

"Carol, this is Lois."

Beep, Be-e-e-p, Be-e-e-e-p. Over the phone I could hear her pager going off. "Oh no," she said. "I'm getting paged."

"I'll hang up and call you back in five minutes," I said. "If it's an emergency and you're gone, I'll just call back later. Bye."

That was typical of our relationship. We would be having lunch and *B-e-e-p*, "Paging number twenty-one." She would have to go stitch up a cut finger. Or tea and pie after Sunday night church and *B-e-e-e-p.* Off she would go to check on a high fever.

"Do you have to go?" I asked when I called five minutes later.

"Yes, but we can talk a minute," she said.

OK, I thought, *Lois, say it out loud. Practice putting your tongue around the word m-a-l-i-g-n-a-n-t.*
. . .

"Carol, I don't want to tell you this, but you're my friend, so you're elected. My mammogram showed a tumor on my left breast."

There was silence on the other end. I knew Carol-my-friend and Carol-the-doctor-person were trying to connect and cope.

"It looks malignant (*There, I said it!*), but we, of course, won't know for sure until Monday."

"Monday?"

"Yes, I told the doctor—by the way, I now have two doctors and this was the surgeon-doctor—anyway, I told him let's just get this show on the road. I couldn't see any sense waiting. He'll do a lumpectomy (That word also stumbled around my tongue before I spit it out.) on Monday if they can work me in."

"What can I do?" Her voice trembled and broke as she spoke.

Dear God, I breathed another "Help, Lord" prayer. *Please help my friends and my family to deal with this. Strengthen them. Give them courage as You have with me and Robert already. Amen.*

"Pray," I said. "I have to call my folks and the boys. Pray for them. I'll call you as soon as we get home tomorrow night. I know you have to go. Love you."

I knew the storm was now over Colstrip. But I also knew that there was a heartfelt prayer winding up through the clouds to the King of all creation. I knew He would calm the waves just as He did for the disciples on the Sea of Galilee.

That verse went through my mind, "Jesus Christ the same yesterday, and today, and for ever" (Hebrews 13:8, KJV). He could control the weather, both outside and inside of me, my family and my friends. *Thank You, Lord.*

Within the next half hour the storm spread.

To Seattle, where our middle son, Kevin, and his wife Kelli live. At times like this, I knew they wished they lived closer to us.

To Glendive, in eastern Montana, where our youngest son Ross and his wife Marla had been living for nearly a year. Then back to Colstrip, where our eldest son Todd, his wife Lisa and our two-year-old grandson Justin live. The clouds were beginning to close in.

Then the hardest call. My folks. They are ranchers in western Montana. I have been a parent for almost thirty years. One fact is certain: No matter how old your kids are and how far away from you they go, that invisible umbilical cord is still there.

Their "kid" was forty-nine years old. She had been away from home a long time, but that was not going to make their pain and caring less. But I could smile as I dialed their number. They trust God. They taught me to trust God. Even in this I know He will be before them. He will provide shelter over them. They will trust Him who is worthy of our trust.

"Mom, hello, how are you?" (After four calls the words still were getting caught in my mouth and swimming around my teeth.) "Can you get Dad on the phone too?"

My mom always says, "What's up?" and she did it again. It must be one of those motherhood-premonition things.

"Well, we've got a little storm here. . . ." Talking to Mom about anything serious always puts a lump in my throat. No matter how old I get. She is still the mother, and I am still the child.

"What are you going to do now?" my mom asked after we had gone over every detail of the forecast.

"Go out and eat and have a wonderful evening together is the main plan. Tomorrow I'm going to the ladies retreat here. Robert is going to canvas the junkyards. Then we'll go home tomorrow night. I want the elders to pray for me. But I also need to do some shopping. I need to get a robe for the hospital."

"Don't get a pink flowered thing. Get something bright and bold. It will make you feel better. And remember we'll be praying."

Months later when we went over our feelings on this day, I learned what a test of faith this was for my parents. They could not believe God would allow this to happen. Their minds did a cancer roll call also. The thoughts of losing their daughter to cancer rained on through the night with thunder and lightning.

Robert and I had had three or four hours to get used to the idea of a weather change ahead. To our dear ones we were calling, the storm had just hit.

"Now what?" Robert has been conditioned over the years to my scheduling and notebook mentality. Whenever we made trips to Billings, there was a list and a schedule. He knew, cancer or not, there would still be a list!

"Well, what do you think about this? Let's go to Hennessys in the mall. I think they'll still be open. I'd like to get a robe and pajamas for the hospital."

I changed into my new blue skirt, red blouse and white linen jacket. This was still *our* night together. Rain clouds or not. Robert dressed up too. We held each other close before we opened the motel room door. We didn't know we were about to see an angel. . . .

At Hennessys, a nice department store in Rimrock Mall, the sunshine broke through the clouds—and it wasn't just because they were having a sale on sleepwear.

There were racks and racks to choose from. I had to look at every one on every rack. Robert was never more than ten inches away. He was already quietly slipping on his own robe—one of caregiver.

My favorite was a Victorian-style cotton robe

with pink flowers intertwined with lace and tiny rosebuds at the neck. I can't help it. I love feminine things.

"You wouldn't know I once taught sewing lessons," I said. "My nightgown at home just needs the neckline mended . . . and new elastic around the cuffs . . . which it has needed for six months!" I laughed as I turned to the man who was now firmly holding an invisible leash made of love and concern. I could feel the constraint as real as if a golden cord was wrapped around my wrist.

He laughed too. "Just buy what you need."

I knew he was thinking about his blue pants pocket! I hung the white and pink robe over my arm.

"I'll carry that for you," he said.

I found pink pajamas. Just because this surgery was going to be on my top, I wasn't baring my bottom half!

He took them too.

Then I saw this bright scarlet robe with two wild green and purple curved stripes down the front. "I need that one too . . . for Mom!"

Robert laid the garments on the counter.

An attractive, poised woman, a little past middle age, was at the cash register. "Oh, looks like you're really taking advantage of our sale," she said and smiled.

"Not really," I confessed. "I'm going into the hospital. It was either mend or buy new—I chose to buy new!"

"Oh, that's not good. Are you going to have surgery?"

Practice, Lois. Say it. "I am going in for a breast biopsy." I thought it was OK to say *breast* since we were standing among the underpants and brassieres.

"Oh, you are? I know all about that."

And right there in the middle of the lingerie department with shoppers mingling around the racks of clothing . . . right there with piped-in music and neon signs beckoning shoppers . . . the sun broke through the clouds. I think I even felt a warm breeze.

"I had breast cancer twelve years ago," she said.

She had our attention.

"First, I got a malignant tumor in my left breast. I had that removed, and then a year later, I had to have my right breast removed."

I looked around. Was she real? Or was she an angel sent from God? Did God put angels on clerk duty at Hennessys? She was real. She was beautiful. She didn't have wings, but she had hair.

"I went through two tough sessions of chemotherapy. I lost all of my hair."

"You look wonderful," I said.

"It hardly seems like it all happened now. I had some tough times with some of the side effects. But now I very seldom think about it." She glanced behind her. Another customer had come up to the counter.

"I hope everything goes well for you too," she said as she put my purchases into a grey Hennessys' bag. "If you can just wait a minute, I'll get you a card. I know a gal that does a great job with wigs. And we have a lady here that works with breast forms and all. . . ."

We waited, in the sunshine, while she finished with the woman across the counter.

I took the cards and put them in my notebook. The wig card and the breast-form business I could deal with later. Right now I wanted to shout to the rooftops: *She's alive!! She had breast cancer twelve years ago . . . and she's alive!!*

Instead I just whispered to Robert, "Now was that from God or what?"

"That definitely was from God," he confirmed.

We walked out of the store, hand in hand. In the sunshine. No, in the *Son*-shine. God was already showing us He knew the whole path of the storm. He was with us.

You can call it a coincidence if you want. Robert and I thanked God that at that time and in that place He sent an angel to us. There was a break in the clouds. Our little finite minds were playing a losing game of hopscotch with our mental cancer roll call. God was showing us the list of survivors.

We arrived at the Jade Palace, a beautifully decorated Chinese restaurant, at peace. God was definitely letting the Son-shine through.

The clouds were lifting. A warm breeze sifted through the night air.

A perfect night for a romantic evening for two. Even three. Robert, me and an angel.

For the moment cancer seemed to slip away.

Weather Forecast—Application

1. In God's Word there are many references to storms and trials in life.

2. Pick up your Bible. Start with the verses listed below. Mark them with a yellow highlighter (Son-shine).

3. Then check your concordance and find others. You can pray that God will lead you to the verses just for you.

4. Watch the sky. Look around you. Be on the lookout for a break in the clouds. Look up. You might miss calming weather if you keep looking down.

Bible References

Weather-related verses:

Psalm 46:1-3	Psalm 18:2
Nahum 1:7	Psalm 37:39
Psalm 118	John 16:33
Psalm 91	Isaiah 43:2

Chapter 4

Living . . . and Dying

In the middle of the night when it was dark, when there was no light, when everyone else was asleep, my thoughts kept me awake:

> *Your friend Pat*
> *just had a small breast tumor*
> *and then she died.*

> *Look what*
> *a good man Dr. Neilson was.*
> *He knew God was going*
> *to heal him. He is in*
> *heaven now.*

> *This is*
> *just what*
> *you deserve. God is punishing you.*

> *The wheelchair in the*
> *grocery store.*

The wheelchair.
Over and over and over . . .

See friend Pat in the wheelchair
being pushed through the grocery store,
so weak,
so bloated,
so sick . . .

Stop!!   Stop!!   Stop!!
. . . radiation, no hair . . .
Stop!!   Stop!!
chemotherapy . . . throwing up . . .
Stop!! In the name of Jesus, stop!!

In the middle of the night. The regular breathing of Robert, sound asleep, is even depressing. Alone. No, I am not alone. Cancer, my uninvited guest, is having a picnic in my body.

———

"See how elusive we are. We don't even
have to advertise. We just come in and
make ourselves at home.
"You don't even know where we are.
Do you suppose we're just in your breast?
Da da da de dah . . .
"That's for us to know and you to find
out. . . ."

———

Oh Lord God, please come to my rescue. I'm in
trouble. My enemies are playing with my mind. Oh

Lord, I don't think I'm qualified for this job You have for me. . . . I'm not worthy. . . . There is sin in my life, Lord. You know it, and I know it. There are things that I don't have victory over.

The still, small voice of the Holy Spirit said, "No, Lois, you are not worthy."

My mind turned into a courtroom. I was both judge and jury. Death could be on the agenda. There was a pile of incriminating evidence on the table between me and my lawyer, my advocate.

The evidence was sin. Unconfessed. Cords of bondage in certain areas. Pleasure of sin enjoyed for the moment. The sin-stack got higher and higher as I looked at myself standing before God. I am a Christian. I love the Lord. I know that when I asked Him to come into my life, years ago, He forgave me my sins.

I knew God's promises:

—"That if thou shalt confess with thy mouth the Lord Jesus, and shalt believe in thine heart that God hath raised him from the dead, thou shalt be saved" (Romans 10:9, KJV).

—"For I will forgive their wickedness and will remember their sins no more" (Hebrews (8:12, NIV).

—"As far as the east is from the west, so far has he removed our transgressions from us" Psalm 103:12, NIV).

I knew beyond a shadow of doubt that if I should die, I would go immediately into the presence of the Lord. That's exactly what was causing me to toss and turn. I didn't want to go into His holy presence with unconfessed sin on my hands.

I stood in the courtroom of my mind, guilty. Guilty of hanging on to some unforgiveness. Guilty of lying. Not a big lie. Just a little "white" lie, just a little stretching of the truth. But in this courtroom, facts are facts and a lie is a lie. I went through the sin-stack on the table. Pride. Lust. Envy. Anger. Fluffy little invisible-to-others things in daintily wrapped containers. Covered with pretty, flowered paper and wrapped with lace . . . until now.

I got out of bed and on my knees.

Oh God, have mercy on me, I prayed through my tears. *I can't deal with cancer in my body until I have dealt with the cancer in my soul. I need Your forgiveness. I need Your cleansing. I've been hanging onto things that aren't pure. Some of these things have wrapped cords of bondage around my soul. Oh Lord God, my heavenly Father, I need You to cleanse me. I need Your mercy.*

And for a long time, in the dark of the night, on my knees in the glaring light of my soul's courtroom, I put the sin-stack under the blood of Jesus Christ. One by one I laid them before my lawyer. My advocate.

And it took a long time. A precious long time. A cleansing long time. The light of dawn was breaking through the motel room curtains as Light was breaking through my soul.

Purifying.
  Healing.
    Mending.
      Forgiving. Filling with mercy.

The sun was up. Night had slunk away. *OK, Cancer, let me see your face. I'm ready. I have already experienced victory because of Christ. And this is just the beginning.*

Living and Dying—Application

My friend John Williams, who had bone cancer four years ago, told me, "Lois, you will think a lot about dying. At least I did."

We do have to think about dying. We have to acknowledge that cancer has just made an invasion. And cancer can be deadly. I just wish we would have this same mind-set without having some possible terminal illness. We do not know the outcome of every day. Only God knows.

In the newspaper we read about the accidental deaths of young and old. There is no warning in many cases. One moment they're here, the next moment they're meeting God, who will say, "Welcome my child" or "Depart from Me, I never knew you."

So we with the invasion of cancer are blessed. We have just been made aware of how fragile life is. Let us use that knowledge wisely.

When you are vulnerable, the enemy, Satan, can use this time in your life to plant discouragement, condemnation, guilt and accusation into your mind.

1. Deal with any past sins as they come to your mind. Then believe that God has forgiven you as He has promised. (See 1 John 1:9.) If the same things keep coming like fiery darts over and over again, consider them from the enemy. Ask God to defeat Satan's attempt to discourage you.

2. Sometimes it helps to write your prayers of confession to the Lord. Then, as one of my friends said, "I just flush that paper down the toilet. It helps me to know they're gone!" Or you could burn it in the fireplace.

3. If you just cannot get victory, go to your pastor or a Christian "saint" you trust. Ask them to pray with you.

4. God never intended us to live under a burden of sin. That is exactly why He sent His Son, Jesus, to die on the cross and rise again to defeat death and sin. "For God hath not given us the spirit of fear; but of power, and of love, and of a sound mind" (2 Timothy 1:7, KJV).

5. Thank God for His mercy and forgiveness! Recognize the fathomless love God has for

you. Read and sing His praises throughout the day. I write verses on recipe cards (since I never use them for recipes!) and carry them in my pocket to read at a stop light or while waiting for an appointment.

Bible References

Psalm 23:4

Psalm 48:14

Psalm 119:65-72

Matthew 6:14

Mark 11:25

John 3:16-17

Romans 3:23

Romans 8:38-39

1 John 1:9

Chapter 5

Meeting Jehoshaphat

"Honey, have you seen my black belt?"
"Mom, where is my algebra book?"
"Kevin, where did you put the car keys?"
"Hey, who had the remote control last?"
Looking. Searching. Seeking. We do it all the time.

A rough week at work doesn't begin to describe my frustration over my job recently. I was behind in finishing many routine tasks. It seemed every time I had a few minutes, someone else made demands on my time. When I did get started on a report or began work on a summary, it took twice as long as it should have.

Tossing and turning at night with job-related situations on my mind and not wanting to get out of bed in the morning were clues that I was in trouble. Three days of this was taking a toll. I woke up on the fourth morning. *Drats! Another day of three steps forward, two steps back.*

Wait! Stop! You dumb bunny! I said to myself. I really couldn't believe it! I hadn't even thought about praying about this situation.

Lord, You must think I am a real ditz! I can pray about cancer and ask You to guide and direct every part of my treatment—but I forgot to pray about my job. Instead I worried and stewed and got more frustrated and You were there all the time . . . waiting for me to ask for Your help.

I felt so stupid. I had not even searched my Bible. I had not prayed about my job problem. We—I—need His help and intervention to live peacefully with ourselves and each other. I just forgot to seek Him.

Looking. Searching. Seeking.

But sometimes we forget where to search.

I knew where to look, to search for answers, for strength and comfort. There was not a doubt in my mind, because I have been through rough times before. The Bible is God's Word. He speaks to us through His Word.

I just forgot.

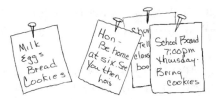

We leave notes on the desk in the kitchen. Or we tape them to the back of the front door. We write notes. We want to communicate with someone who we cannot call or won't be seeing right away. We want them to read the note or we wouldn't have written it.

God inspired His chosen writers to put down "instructions" for us, not to be ignored, but to be read. He knew we needed comfort and direction, instructions and guidance.

✳   ✳   ✳

It was Saturday night. A little over twenty-four hours since the "Cancer Recruiter" had called my number. I sat on the bed with my Bible on my lap. *Lord, I need Your guidance. I'm seeking Your direction for this path I'm about to walk. I am coming to You. In Jesus' name, amen.*

---

*"Lump . . . tumor . . . surgery . . .
tumor . . . cancer . . . malignant . . .
chemotherapy . . radiation . . . surgery."*

"Listen to me. . . . The Lᴏʀᴅ is with you when you are with him. If you seek him, he will be found by you . . ." (2 Chronicles 15:2, NIV).

"But if from thence thou shalt seek the Lᴏʀᴅ thy God, thou shalt find *him*, if thou seek him with all thy heart and with all thy soul" (Deuteronomy 4:29, KJV).

"But seek first his kingdom and his righteousness, and all these things will be given to you as well" (Matthew 6:33, NIV).

Notice each verse says, "If you seek Him" . . . "If thou shalt seek the Lord". . . "But seek first."

"Tumor . . . cancer . . . radiation . . . chemotherapy."

Opening my Bible, I thumbed through the pages. Waiting. Listening. Seeking for something to jump off the pages. Searching for God's message to me. This is what I found.

God's Word can stand on its own. It does not need my interpretation. First, I want you to read this chapter. Let it speak to you. Following the passage from Second Chronicles, I will describe how God ministered to me and laid out the whole path in front of me . . . from His Word.

2 Chronicles 20:1-30 (KJV)

It came to pass after this also, that the children of Moab, and the children of Ammon, and with them other beside the Ammonites, came against Jehoshaphat to battle. Then there came some that told Jehoshaphat, saying, There cometh a great multitude against thee from beyond the sea on this side Syria; and, behold, they be in Hazazon-tamar, which is Engedi. And Jehoshaphat feared, and set himself to seek the LORD, and proclaimed a fast throughout all Judah. And Judah gathered themselves together, to ask help of the LORD: even out of all the cities of Judah they came to seek the LORD. And Jehoshaphat stood in the congregation of Judah and Jerusalem, in the house of LORD, before the new court. And said,

O LORD God of our fathers, art not thou God in heaven? and rulest not thou over all the kingdoms of the heathen? and in thine hand is there not power and might, so that none is able to withstand thee? Art not thou our God, who didst drive out the inhabitants of this land before thy people Israel, and gavest it to the seed of Abraham thy friend for ever? And they dwelt therein, and have built thee a sanctuary therein for thy name, saying, If, when evil cometh upon us, as the sword, judgment, or pestilence, or famine, we stand before this house, and in thy presence, (for thy name is in this house,) and cry unto thee in our affliction, then thou wilt hear and help. And now, behold, the children of Ammon and Moab and mount Seir, whom thou wouldest not let Israel invade, when they came out of the land of Egypt, but they turned from them, and destroyed them not; Behold, I say, how they reward us, to come to cast us out of thy possession, which thou hast given us to inherit. O our God, wilt thou not judge them? for we have no might against this great company that cometh against us; neither know we what to do: but our eyes are upon thee.

And all Judah stood before the LORD, with their little ones, their wives, and their children.

Then upon Jahaziel the son of Zechariah, the son of Benaiah, the son of Jeiel, the son of Mattaniah, a Levite of the sons of Asaph, came the Spirit of the LORD in the midst of the congregation;

And he said, Hearken ye, all Judah, and ye inhabitants of Jerusalem, and thou king Jehoshaphat, Thus saith the LORD unto you, Be not afraid nor dismayed by reason of this great multitude; for the battle is not yours, but God's. To morrow go ye down against them: behold, they come up by the cliff of Ziz; and ye shall find them at the end of the brook, before the wilderness of Jeruel. Ye shall not need to fight in this battle: set yourselves, stand ye still, and see the salvation of the LORD with you, O Judah and Jerusalem: fear not, nor be dismayed; to morrow go out against them: for the LORD will be with you.

And Jehoshaphat bowed his head with his face to the ground: and all Judah and the inhabitants of Jerusalem fell before the LORD, worshipping the LORD. And the Levites, of the children of the Kohathites, and of the children of the Korhites, stood up to praise the LORD God of Israel with a loud voice on high.

And they rose early in the morning, and went forth into the wilderness of Tekoa: and as they went forth, Jehoshaphat stood and said, Hear me, O Judah, and ye inhabitants of Jerusalem; Believe in the LORD your God, so shall ye be established; believe his prophets, so shall ye prosper. And when he had consulted with the people, he appointed singers unto the LORD, and that should praise the beauty of holiness, as they went out before the army, and to say, Praise the LORD; for his mercy endureth for ever. And when they began to sing and to praise, the LORD set ambushments against the children of Ammon, Moab, and mount Seir, which were come against Judah; and they were smitten. For the children of Ammon and Moab stood up against the inhabitants of mount Seir, utterly to slay and destroy them: and when they had made an end of the inhabitants of Seir, every one helped to destroy another.

And when Judah came toward the watch tower in the wilderness, they looked unto the multitude, and, behold, they were dead bodies fallen to the earth, and none escaped. And when Jehoshaphat and his people came to take away the spoil of them, they found among them in abundance both riches with the dead bodies, and precious jewels, which they stripped off for themselves, more than they could carry away: and they were three days in gathering of the spoil, it was so much. And on the fourth day they assembled themselves in the valley of Berachah; for there they blessed the Lord: therefore the name of the same place was called, The valley of Berachah, unto this day.

Then they returned, every man of Judah and Jerusalem, and Jehoshaphat in the forefront of them, to go again to Jerusalem with joy; for the Lord had made them to rejoice over their enemies. And they came to Jerusalem with psalteries and harps and trumpets unto the house of the Lord.

And the fear of God was on all the

kingdoms of those countries, when they had heard that the LORD fought against the enemies of Israel. So the realm of Jehoshaphat was quiet: for his God gave him rest round about.

*   *   *

Remember?

If you seek him, he will be found by you (2 Chronicles 15:2 NIV).

I met Jehoshaphat and I found Him—God.

I found direction. I found comfort and courage. I found strength and hope. I found how to *live victoriously* with cancer.

Words cannot adequately describe to you how overwhelmed I felt as I sat on that bed with my Bible open on my lap. God had spoken. He had a plan. For me.

I felt an immediate call to battle. As sure as if Uncle Sam had laid his hand on my shoulder and said, "Lois, there is going to be a war. Grab your boots and get your uniform. Here is your battle plan."

Only it wasn't Uncle Sam. It was God. It wasn't make-believe. It was cancer. It was me . . . and Jehoshaphat.

Let me share with you the plan that was unfolded in front of me through this chapter.

Verse 1—There was going to be a battle.

This was not just a "little valley" in my Christian walk. I needed to grab my helmet, shield and sword. The enemy was already "in" and the battle lines were set. From this moment forth, I would fight. I prepared my heart and my mind for the battle.

Verse 3—He sought the Lord.

Along with Jehoshaphat, I set myself to seek the Lord. I called upon the Lord. I was seeking His guidance through His holy Word.

Verse 4—They gathered themselves to ask help of the LORD.

I knew I was not to keep silent. I called my family and friends. We set prayer chains in motion. Many churches were called for prayer support. At least thirty churches, with various doctrines and from all over the country, prayed for us weekly throughout treatment. We met with our pastor immediately. We called upon the elders according to James 5:14. They anointed me with oil and prayed for me. God may also call you to fast and pray.

Verse 6—O LORD God of our fathers.

I knew I could trust my Lord, Jehoshaphat's Lord. *The Lord God is trustworthy.* He was reminding me.

Verse 9—We cry unto Thee in our affliction.

I trust this ministers to you also. Wherever you are, with financial difficulties or marriage problems, cry unto the Lord. If you have cancer, or one you love has cancer, we can cry unto our Lord. I did. Robert did. My family did.

Verse 10—The enemies are invading.

And it was an invasion. Cancer was invading my body. The enemy had already stealthily crept over the walls. My blood veins and bone marrow were tunnels for their battalions. They were setting up base camps and preparing to spread out.

Verse 12—We have no might against this great company that comes against us.

I couldn't agree more. *Without Thee, O Lord, we are helpless. We just so often forget. Help me remember!*

Verse 12—But our eyes are upon Thee!

I prayed, *Lord, keep my eyes ever and continually on Thee. I want to be focused on Thee. Not on the circumstances.*

Verse 15—Be not afraid nor dismayed.

What comfort and courage and peace from this verse. I repeated it over and over. It became my battle cry. It kept me during wakeful nights. It gleamed in neon colors in my brain during radiation and chemotherapy.

"Be not afraid nor dismayed by reason of
this great multitude
[of cancer cells];
for the battle is not yours, but God's."

Immediately my focus was off the enemy, the cancer, and onto my army general, commander in chief—Jesus!

Verse 17—You shall have no need to fight in this battle . . .

Set yourselves. . . . Stand still. . . . See the salvation of the Lord *with you!*

Again and again when I wanted to activate, push, stew or pressure the doctors, my family or God, I was reminded of this verse. Hundreds of times when circumstances were not what I wanted them to be, I heard that quiet voice of the Holy Spirit repeating this verse to me. I am a do-er, a fixer, an in-charge personality. This was probably one of my harder lessons. God constantly brought this verse to mind. I believe it will be with me through my life as a positive goal. Praise God. Another miracle within the battle.

Verse 17—Fear not nor be dismayed.

By His mercy and with His strength, fear was not a constant companion. There were attacks of fear that I recognized immediately and dealt with them as if in warfare. Others were subtle. But an overall fear for my life was dealt with through God's promises and

His direction, "Do not fear." God is able. What a promise!

Verse 17—For the Lord will be with you.

I wrote this book as evidence. Hear my testimony. In living with cancer and in dying with cancer, God is there—if you invite Him, as your Lord and Savior, to be there. I accepted this promise and knew it would be as written.

Verse 20—Believe in the LORD your God, so shall you be established.

I believe in God's ability to heal. I also believe we are healed in different ways. How could I explain that to others? Then I saw the word "established."

That was the desire of my heart, regardless of the cancer, to be "established" with the Lord. Read Webster's definition:

> *es-tab-lish*, v. l: to make firm or stable 2: to institute permanently by enactment or agreement
> 3: to settle 4: to bring into existence (found)
> 5: to set on a firm basis 6: to put beyond doubt or prove.

Verse 21—He appointed singers that they should praise.

This verse became my precept, my modus operandi. I felt directed as surely as if I had been handed a written order from God saying, "Sing, Lois."

I can't sing. I really cannot sing. My family will bear witness, as well as those who sit beside me in church! When I was young, I got nickels for being quiet. But I determined to sing in the weeks ahead because God told me to. I would just sing quietly.

Verse 22—And when . . .

Faith follows action. Sing and trust. Sing and believe. Sing and see the ambushment built. Watch.

Verse 22—They were smitten.

You know the "they" in my mind!

"So you're replacing the defense with the offense? We can handle that. No problem. We'll rewrite Act two!"

Chapter 6

Prepping for Surgery . . . Do I Need Gloves?

I felt such peace. Robert and I made a before church appointment with Pastor Mike.

"What's up?" he asked as we sat down in his study early Sunday morning.

"Lois is going in for surgery in the morning," Robert said. "She has to have a biopsy."

I was finding it easier to say "breast" out loud. Robert was not. We sure had had a lot of practice since Friday.

"I have a tumor in my left breast, and it could be malignant," I said. "The doctor thinks it is."

Shock and concern showed in his eyes. I like this young pastor. I didn't at first because I didn't think he was very compassionate. But with God's prompting I began to notice the small, tenderhearted ways about him. We have a good relationship now. And he was kind to me.

"What can we do?" he asked. He came, sat right next to me and put his hand on mine.

"I take James 5:14 literally," I said. "It says if there are any sick among you, 'let him call for the elders of the church; and let them pray over him, anointing him with oil in the name of the Lord.' I want to do that this morning."

Pastor Mike agreed. He asked about the arrangements we had made for the next day. He offered any assistance we might need. He asked two more questions before he bowed his head to pray with us.

"Bob, how are you doing with all this?"

Mentally I said, *Thanks, God, for this young man, this compassionate (!) young man.*

Robert grabbed onto my shoulder and looked at the pastor, "I'll be fine."

Next the pastor asked if I felt like leading the worship service as I usually did. It was about time to begin the service.

"Of course," I said.

He prayed for us. Then he said, "I'll call the elders up to the front altar after the service. We will anoint you with oil and pray. What do you want to say? Do you want to tell them what's going on?"

"No, I want you to tell them," I said. "I might get teary because I know it will be hard for them. These church people are my family. I know the depth of their love for us. I want them to know it all so they will know how to pray." (I also thought, *It will be a test to see if he can say "breast" out loud!*)

We left his study assured that he would be

walking this path with us. I hurried to the church kitchen where I knew I would find my friend Phyllis, a soul mate and dear sister in the Lord.

"I need to tell you something," I said, "and Jim too."

Her husband poured coffee into my mug. We have mug racks on the wall in our church kitchen. Everyone has a favorite personal mug hanging there. He poured coffee for himself and Phyllis and then stood beside me. In a few sentences I shared my news. Her arms were around me before I finished.

"We will pray," they both said. I knew they would. They had been through some tough times. They were sturdy prayer warriors.

Then I looked for Pete. I needed to find my friend Pete and tell him too. Our bond was a special one. He had ministered to me, as I had to him, many times in the past. He wasn't in his Sunday school room to teach yet. I couldn't find him. As I headed back to the sanctuary, my eye caught Phyllis and Jim in an empty classroom. Her head was on Jim's shoulder, and she was crying.

Pastor Mike finished his sermon, of which I cannot remember a word. Then he said, "Before we leave today I want the elders to come."

He went on to explain about the tumor and the surgery the next day. I felt such peace and confidence knowing I was doing what God had instructed. Whatever happened the next day and the next and in the weeks ahead was in God's hands. I was doing my part in obedience. The rest was totally in His control.

As I sat in front of the church on a chair, with Robert beside me, I quietly confessed all of the sins that came to my mind so that I would be offering a clean vessel for God's healing.

Pastor Mike and the elders, including Pete and Jim, gathered around us. My heart went out to Pete. I could see the grief on his face.

Pastor Mike read the verses again as he dipped his fingers into the oil and touched my forehead. "Is any sick among you? let him call for the elders of the church; and let them pray over him, anointing him with oil in the name of the Lord: And the prayer of faith shall save the sick, and the Lord shall raise him up; and if he have committed sins, they shall be forgiven him" (James 5:14-15, KJV).

What a joy to know if I forgot one or more, those sins would be forgiven too! As I thanked the Lord I knew beyond a shadow of doubt that my future was secure in His will.

How He chose to heal me, by a touch of His hand, by the touch of His hand on the doctors' hands or by taking me to heaven, I felt calm and at perfect peace.

———————

"Well, we could have done without that! We've dealt with praying people before. Like you're the first Christian with cancer?

The first person to pray? No way! It's just an inconvenience, that's all. We'll deal with it."

By Sunday night "Lois' news" was out in Colstrip. We packed our bags and drove back to Billings. When we got to our motel, I peeled off my fake fingernails. It would be embarrassing if one or two came unglued in surgery. That might cause some panic in the operating room.

*   *   *

"How did you get your fingernails so long?" I asked my friend.

My fingernails always show the effects of typing, wallpapering and other sundry household duties. When dressing up for a special occasion I often wished gloves were back in style.

"It's a secret," she said. But then in a display of true friendship, she went on. "I get them at Target for $2.97. You just glue them on."

Well, I have never been one to deny vanity. We were making plans for an overnight trip to the city. Fingernails for Lois were on our list.

It was like slipping back into high school days! We sat on the bed in our hotel room. All the necessary equipment spread around us to launch my fingers on their beauty trip. Sharon was a seasoned pro. Soon I was practicing dialing the phone and fastening buttons with my fake finery. Oh, how feminine I felt! Pink frosted nail polish. Clear lacquer top coat. That was several months ago.

Now I'm a pro also. The great thing I learned is that after a few weeks with the plastic cover job, my own nails grow. Then I take the fake ones off, and I have real long nails of my own. Sounds terrific, doesn't it? Femininity at the low, low price of $2.97. However, to all good deals there are a few drawbacks. In this case, it is the glue. I imagine the reason nail salons charge more is because they spend a bit more on the fastening factor. But I can put up with a few drawbacks, like occasionally, one of my glamorous nails flies off.

A few weeks ago, we were just beginning our main course at a Christian Women's Club dinner. I picked up my fork, and it slid out of my hand. It caught my ring finger, my nail to be exact.

Karen was sitting across from me. She flinched and said, "What was that??"

The lady next to her said, "I don't know. Something just flew by my face!"

Now the cheap-nail-owner dilemma: Do I say "Oh, that was my fingernail"? Or do I just keep my now stark white, stubby ring finger curled in hiding during dinner?

I 'fessed up, retrieved the bright pink nail, quickly getting my handy-dandy, repair glue bottle from my purse. Everyone at the table was very interested in the procedure!

My husband swears if I ever get lost, he will just follow my trail of fingernails until I'm found.

But the worst disaster happened at work. It was the end of the month. We were doing the monthly billing. I had stuffed about 300 envelopes when I discovered one of my nails was missing. I frantically searched the area. My co-workers wondered why I was so prudently going over each envelope, carefully sealing the flap. Actually I was trying to feel for a fingernail. I didn't find the elusive little bugger.

All I could do was pray. *Dear Lord, please don't let some customer come to my desk next week and tell me there was a fingernail in their bill.*

I did establish a backup plan in case the Lord said "No" to my plea. "We planted some of these nails in our bills," I would say. "It's an advertising tool. Did you know you can buy these great little items for only $2.97 at Target?"

On second thought, maybe you just better try the professional ones!

✳ ✳ ✳

The afternoon in Colstrip had been spent packing and making more phone calls to co-workers and friends. We were so comforted by their concern. By the time we checked into our motel room, we were both tired.

My mom came from Livingston to be with us. Todd and Lisa and my Dad would come in the morning. Carol was there Sunday night too. Her love was evidenced by all the arrangements necessary for her to be with me. Another health care provider had to be found to take her place at the clinic in Colstrip.

I wrote in my journal: "Feel wonderful and no sense of fear or worry. Outcome is in God's hands and I do not doubt Him!"

I slept well. I don't think Robert did.

Love was surrounding me. I was touched again with humbleness when my mom gave me a small, gift-wrapped box in the morning. Inside were tiny glistening Black Hills gold earrings.

"Well, without your makeup and fingernails, I thought you needed something!" she joked.

We hugged again and left for the clinic. A chest X-ray was scheduled for 9 a.m. Marcia Hully, a friend for years, was the technician. *Thank You, Lord.*

Her mother-in-law had breast cancer two years before and was doing well, she told me. "Dennis and I will be praying for you," she said when she finished the medical procedure.

Dr. Brown's nurse, Lisa, called us in.

"I have scheduled your surgery for noon," said Dr. Brown as he sat down. "Now what questions do you have?"

Breathing a quick *Thank You, Lord, for a caring doctor*, I said, "I forgot to ask you what it is going to look like?" He knew "it" was the breast-word.

He pulled his pen out of his shirt pocket and drew a circle on the exam table paper cover. "Here is your breast. Here is the location of the lump. I will make an incision right here about an inch above the nipple." He went on to describe how he would remove the lump and a small rim of surrounding tissue. The lump would immediately be sent to pathology. If the tests showed any malignancy, he would remove the lymph nodes under my arm to see if the cancer had spread. He went over the consent forms, and I signed my name.

"Are you sure there are no more questions?" he asked.

I glanced at Robert, and he shook his head.

Dr. Brown shook Robert's hand and patted mine. "I'll see you at noon," he said.

I left the room thinking . . . *for lunch, I believe I'll have a lumpectomy.*

We had an hour before I had to check in at the hospital. I felt like a celebrity with an entourage; Robert, Mom, Dad, Todd, Lisa and Carol were with me every step. So were my cancer cells . . . but I didn't know it yet.

Robert held the hospital door open. I walked through, followed by Mom, Dad, Todd, Lisa, Carol and then Robert. We were lined up like my ducks coming in for feeding time. Their presence was love-filled. Conversation was trivial. No one said the *C* word.

"If *this* turns out to be nothing, we'll eat at

Gusicks," I told Dad. It was his favorite place to eat, our least favorite.

"And I'll buy!" he said.

Robert and I stepped up to the admitting desk.

"What can I do for you?" said the pretty woman with the keys (the computer ones) to enter the medical kingdom.

"I'm Lois Olmstead. I am having surgery for lunch."

"Could you spell that?"

"L-u-n-c-h."

With one glance I could tell humor was not appropriate.

"Oh, L-o-i-s O-l-m-s-t-e-a-d."

"Still at 7403 Castle Rock Lake Drive in Colstrip?"

"Yes." *They must be tied in with the FBI, IRS and SSA!*

"You are insured with Blue Cross/Blue Shield?"

"Yes." *Wonder what a "no" answer would change?*

"You are scheduled for outpatient surgery with Dr. Dennis Brown?"

"Yes." *Suppose if it turns out to be more, he'll have to treat me in the street. I just hate the way they kick you out of hospitals now-a-days. I'll probably go home with tubes hanging out of my body!*

"You're all set, Mrs. Olmstead. The nurse will be with you in a few minutes. Have a seat."

"The nurse will be with you in a few minutes. The doctor will be with you in a few minutes. Then in a few minutes they will know we are with you too. Have a seat!"

Everyone patted my hand. I snuggled a little closer to Robert on the burgundy waiting room couch.

"You OK?" I asked for the millionth time.

"Yup, you OK?" he replied for the million-and-first time.

The nurse came out with a clipboard in hand. She surveyed the sitting ducks. There were lots to choose from.

"Mrs. Olmstead?"

"That's me," I said.

Everyone stood up.

"You can all wait here," she said.

Everyone sat down.

"We're just going over her history. I'll take the rest of you to the surgery waiting area in a few minutes."

I went into a little office. Mom followed. (This is a typical hen-step mom. Ain't nobody messin' with her chick without her OK!) I was going to tease her, but the nurse with the clipboard was poised with pen.

"Have you eaten anything this morning?" she asked.

"No." Then the other questions followed:

"Age? Aspirin? Allergic? Anesthesia?"
"Bleeding? Blood Pressure?"
"Coughing? . . . "

I hope we don't have to go through the whole alphabet, I thought. *Nope. Next question—W.*
"Will? Do you have a living will?"
"No. But we're going to do that someday."
"Do you want to sign the papers today?"
"No. But I sure will read the brochure," I promised as she handed one to me.

After going over the risks of surgery and anesthesia and asking if I understood everything, she allowed me to sign in. I didn't have to put down our vehicle license number and when we planned to check out.

She gave me a bracelet with my name and Dr. Brown's name on it. Then I followed her to the day-surgery prep room.

"I want to see my family before I go," I told her.

"They can come in after you get the gown on and get in bed. You can leave your underpants on. Just everything above the waist off."

Life's little blessings. I get to keep my underpants on. Grandma Lennemann was right. She always said, "Wear clean underwear everyday. You never know when you might end up in the hospital!"

We were gearing up for action now. A blood pressure cuff was put on my arm. There was a donation of blood for the lab tech with the tray of bottles. An IV needle was put in my arm.

There were other patients in the assembly-line room. Curtains hung between the beds. Another nurse came in carrying a tray with a syringe and needle thing.

"Is this it?" I asked, clad in a white hospital gown and pink underpants ensemble.

"This will make you drowsy very quickly," she said.

"I want to pray with my family first!"

"They're right out here; I'll get them."

Robert, Mom, Dad, Todd, Lisa and Carol were summoned. They gathered around the bed.

"Mom, you pray," I said. The effectual fervent prayer of a righteous mother-hen availeth much (James 5:16 KJV, freely translated by me).

"Lord, be with Lois right now. Be with this Dr. Brown and all the nurses. Lord, we ask You to just heal her body. In Jesus' name, amen."

I felt hugs from my toes to my neck as each one gave me a squeeze before filing out of the room.

Robert looked into my eyes. "I love you."

"I love you too."

The nurse put the sleepy stuff in my IV. They started pushing my bed down the hall. My little troop of ducks followed. Robert squeezed my hand. Big double doors swung open.

I went somewhere.

"Did I talk? After they gave me that shot? Did I say something?" I asked Todd weeks later.

"Yes, you talked. You talked a mile-a-minute going down the hall. But you didn't say anything . . . as usual," said Todd, my eldest loving son!

Chapter 7

The Operation . . . Was I There?

Robert: It took forever. I didn't think you were ever going to get out of there. The longer it took, the more I knew *it* was cancer.

Dad: I just could not believe this was happening to you. It could have been just a regular day but here we all were in the hospital. I was pretty sure, I guess you told us, it was probably cancer. I just couldn't believe it was you.

Mom: I told God it just could not be cancer. After all the years of struggles and heartache with Ron [my brother] and his cluster headaches, you couldn't have cancer. We had been pleading with God for years to heal those headaches. We just could not have this happen to our other child.

Lisa: I just knew it wasn't going to be cancer. I just knew God was going to make it be nothing.

Todd: I just figured, *Whatever.* I knew we all could handle anything. I figured God would know what He was doing.

Carol: Medical knowledge is a personal handicap when it comes to your friends. Statistics are imprinted in your brain. Finding Robert and Lois as friends when I moved to Colstrip had been a godsend. This just could not be.

The Operating Room Procedure

(Note: This is a "typical" procedure. Each patient and each surgeon may have a slightly different procedure.)

I am told that I had plenty to talk about in the operating room, too. You know me. I never pass up an opportunity for conversation, whether or not anyone else wants to join in. The way I talked in the hall going to the operating room, I wonder how much I didn't really say.

I love the moment before falling asleep, such warmth and peace. I missed it this time. Did I count backward from 100? No dreams, either. Maybe that was just as well. It might have been a nightmare about, you know, C-A-N-C-E-R.

While I slept, my left breast and arm were cleansed with iodine solution. Sky blue drapes covered all of me except for my left chest and arm. Yet another group of strangers to whom I would bare my breast. Dr. Brown made a gently arcing incision over the lump. The incision

was planned to provide enough room to remove the entire lump, yet create a cosmetically
appealing scar. Can there be such a thing on a
breast? More on that later.

The specimen was quickly transported to the
pathology lab while I continued my dreamless
sleep. There, a frozen section was performed
which in fifteen to twenty minutes would provide Dr. Brown with a verdict.

"Denny, we are talking about Lois Olmstead.
This is invasive carcinoma. The margins are
clear," the pathologist reported dryly. The surgeon wants a rim of normal tissue around the
cancer. Otherwise, more breast tissue will be
excised.

With invasive carcinoma, the axilliary, or un-
der-arm, lymph nodes need to be removed.
Lymph nodes filter fluid from the tissues that is
returning to the bloodstream. In the case of the
breast, much of that drains through the axilla.

It takes a day or two to process the results.
Knowing the size of the tumor and whether
the cancer has spread allows the cancer to be
staged. In turn, stage helps determine what additional treatment to undergo.

With the nodes removed, Dr. Brown inserted
a drain under my arm to collect lymph that
would drain for a week or two. Next stop: recovery room . . . then reality.

*   *   *

At 2:37 p.m. Dr. Brown came through the double doors into the waiting room. "It was malignant."

"I remember Carol started crying," Lisa told me later. "I just couldn't believe it was cancer."

Dr. Brown asked if they had any questions. Then he said, "We got all we could see. Now we'll wait for the pathology report. You can see her when she gets out of recovery. She will be in a room down the hall. The nurse will come get you."

"Did you think I was going to die?" I asked Robert about that moment.

"Yes, I figured that might happen. But my next thought was, *We're going to fight this thing.* Together we would fight."

The Recovery Room

No one had to tell me the tumor was malignant. No one had to say "Lois, we have some bad news. You had cancer in that lump in your breast."

With my first fleeting wave of semiconsciousness, I knew the tumor was cancer. I knew because my armpit hurt.

My armpit really hurt!

Like screaming-out-loud, no-pride, help-me pain!

"If the tumor is malignant, I'll take out lymph nodes under your arm so we can check them," Dr. Brown had said that morning.

I have cancer, I thought as I floated off in that soft cushion of fuzzy clouds.

---

*"Hey you, lab tech! How long are we
going to sit crammed in this petri dish?
And where's Lois so we can spread out?
"Ouch! Watch it with that needle,
you big oaf!
"Wait! Before you do that, let us send this
message by c-mail to our old homestead:
'Not tonight, hon. We have headaches.
We don't feel like multiplying.' "*

Robert kept his part of our prearranged agreement. I had said, "When I get out of surgery and back in a room, I want you to turn on my tape deck. Promise?" He promised.

Carefully I had picked tapes of hymns. Old hymns. Hymns that would remind me of God. Spiritual songs that would set my mind on a sure foundation. I knew I wouldn't feel like singing when I came out of surgery. So I would follow my "sing-precept" in this manner.

The hymns were inside a lava lamp. That's where I was. Remember those lamps that look like they have egg yolks of purple, blue, yellow, orange and pink lazily floating in oil? The yolks float up and down, merge and separate, gliding in various slippery shapes. I was a pink yolk.

A hurting pink yolk. I was the victim of a cruel trick. They lied to me. They told me I would get painkillers. I had never had surgery before. Naturally I thought painkillers would kill the pain. Wrong!

They must not have given me any, was my semi conscious conclusion.

"Robert, tell them to give me the painkillers." My words were coming out fuzzy. *It must be the oil in the lamp where I'm swimming.*

Robert was sitting beside my bed.

"Please stay right with me," I had told him the night before. He was. The rest of my fluff-covered family were at the foot of my bed. I shut my eyes so they would think I was asleep. I felt like I was supposed to be part of their conversation. But my brain wasn't sending my words to my mouth.

"On Christ the solid rock I stand . . ."

I can't stand. My yolk keeps floating off the rock. My armpit hurts!

"Robert, they forgot to give me painkillers."

"They didn't forget. They gave you something for pain."

There was talking at the foot of the bed. Evidently the flock of ducks was still following me.

Gary Walker, a cowboy evangelist and friend of my folks, said, "Lois, I've been praying for you. Sorry we have to meet like this. I wanted to be here with your folks."

"Good to meet you," I said.

Maybe the nurse with the pain stuff couldn't get through because there were so many people in the room. When I heard Dad say,

"Maybe we ought to get something to eat?" I jumped on the idea.

"Yes, go get something to eat. *All of you* get something to eat." Probably not very polite, but this was a desperate hour. *I need some painkillers!*

Later when I asked Robert what I did those first few hours, he was honest, "You just kept asking for pain medicine. You kept saying that they didn't give you any!"

After breast surgery you may not have lots of pain. Every woman undergoing breast cancer surgery reacts differently. Some of my friends who are breast cancer survivors spent only one day in the hospital. Some experienced severe pain, some did not. Some got sick, some did not. I didn't have pain in my breast where the incision was made, but *my armpit really hurt.*

"The two areas are different," Dr. Brown explained when he came in. "Under your arm when we cut through the skin, there can be bruising of muscle tissue. Your lymph nodes are tiny glands buried in fatty tissue. I removed some of those nodes. The pain will subside but you will have different sensations around the axillary dissection. Numbness or a tingling feeling is common."

Surprisingly, given the rising and falling, slipping and floating of my pink yolk, I did not feel nauseated. That is . . . until the person in the bed next to me, who I couldn't see because of a curtain between us, started throwing up.

I heard a nurse say, "Honey, just breathe. You had your tonsils out. The hurt will go away."

Yeah, sure, I thought. *They forgot to give her any painstuff too. What is there? A shortage of drugs at this place?*

The floating yolk and the power of suggestion proved to be too great. The next several hours are not polite to write about. I have dismissed them from my memory.

Except for three things:

1. Robert never left my side. I felt love, support and concern in his presence. He lovingly placed his hand on mine or gently touched my face.

2. Dr. Brown came and checked on me. I didn't like him very much at the moment. And I told him about the forgotten painkillers!

3. The words of the hymns ministered to my mind. I was continually reminded that God was with me. He was my strength.

By the next day, I felt better. I got some relief from the armpit pain. I quit throwing up. I even enjoyed the flowers, cards and calls from friends. Visits were special. Each act was a gift from God. I felt so at peace. My future was in the hands of the Potter who molded me of clay.

Another angel from God was Pat Nickel. She came to my bedside with a pair of socks. "I don't want to stay long. I just want to tell you I have been there. I went through what you're going through. You will feel better. God will be with you."

"I have been there. . . ." were the best words my ears heard. *See she had cancer. She is still alive.* The game of cancer roll call was still being played out in my mind. The enemy just lost two points.

I was dismissed from the hospital at 7 p.m. on Wednesday.

- I had a list of directions from the hospital.

- I had a permission slip to go back to work in five days.

- I had a list of arm instructions.

- I had an appointment slip to see Dr. Brown on the 12th.

- I had a note to see Dr. Lamm at the Cancer Center on the 19th.

- I had a tube coming out from my armpit complete with an attached drain bag.

I was right. I would go home with a tube hanging out of me! Stepping from the wheelchair into our car, I looked forward to going home.

So this is what cancer is like, I thought. *It's so weird. I didn't feel it before. I don't feel it now. Weird.*

The two-hour trip went quickly for me.

For Robert it was a different matter. He was my nurse. He went at it like it was a new project that just came into his engineering department. It would be done right! With military precision, medication charts and direct orders—all conceived and carried out with deep loving concern. He knew where the tough places would be. I don't take orders well. Resting does not come easily. (Unless I'm depressed about something, then I want my blankey and bed!)

"We'll let you glide along a while.
We can wait. We have lots of time. . . .
We have the rest of your life."

Robert got me settled in my hovel. It's my favorite room in our house. My desk, computer, books—my stuff is all there. There's a sign on the door:

> *hovel* \\'hov-el,\\ n. [ME] 1: An open shed or shelter 2: Tabernacle 3: A small, wretched and often dirty hut.
>
> Welcome to my hovel . . . may GOD bless you and me as you enter . . .

It was crowded with the bed in the room. But it would be a good place for me to rest, with all of my stuff close by, including a phone. The bathroom was across the hall. Sleeping in our waterbed was out of the question. I certainly did not want to jiggle yet!

Besides, above all, Robert needed to rest also. His face was showing the strain already. I knew this all was going to be harder on him than on me.

Please, Lord, be with Robert. Help him through this. Watch over him. In Jesus' name, amen.

Family and friends showered me with love. It was overwhelming.

> How do I describe being held in the hand of God?
>
> What words can portray the comfort of His staff and rod?
>
> The flood of peace, trust and faith in my soul?
>
> The sweet assurance that He is fully in control?
>
> The Lord is my Shepherd, I shall not fear?
>
> He is leading me, though the path ahead is unclear.
>
> — Anonymous

How many prayers does it take to cure cancer? I have yet to find the answer. But I can testify. The prayers raised on my behalf brought a peace that I had never before experienced.

I wrote in my journal that night:

Two things I know now—I am healed—
as God wills. And I have had my sins forgiven by grace and the promise of God. I
also know of everything I have in this life,
my family and friends are the most precious. The most miraculous occurrence
was how soon it was over. Two days and
I am well on the way to feeling great. I
am so blessed. Thank You, Holy God!

The next day I wrote:

I have to remember, Lord, this is Your
battle. Your miracle does not depend on
how "good" I am, but on Your grace and
mercy and loving kindness—and Your
patience in that we count this earthly life
so dear and You know differently. Patiently let us learn—this world is not our
home. The sole outcome of this all does
not depend on the radiation, the opera-
tion, the doctors, the chemotherapy—it is
Yours, Lord.

I remembered the joke someone told at
church. A flood covered the man's land. The
water was so deep he had to get on his roof. He
was a devoutly religious man. "God," he yelled,
"I believe You will get me off this roof. I will
wait for You." A helicopter came. The man
wouldn't grab the rope. "God is going to rescue
me," he yelled. He gave the same answer to a

rescue boat and a life raft filled with people sent to help him. Soon he was up to his neck in flood waters, losing his grasp on the chimney. "God," he wailed. "Why did You let me down? Why didn't You save me?"

From the heavens he heard the voice of God, "I sent you a helicopter, a rescue boat, a life raft. What did you want?"

Lord, I'm watching. I'll take the helicopter.

All week I rested. People from the church brought meals. Others brought food for the freezer to be taken out as needed. Our neighbors and coworkers were there to lend a hand. The post office box was full of cards.

"God bless friends," Robert said as he sat beside my bed. "The smoke alarm will feel neglected!"

We were eating a delicious meal. (I was not cooking!)

"Did you call Karen yet?" Robert asked.

"No, it's just so hard to hear how this hurts those I love."

"You have to call her. Do it tonight."

Karen is my friend in Texas. She used to live in Colstrip. We had a special bond, both being the mom of three boys.

"Karen, this is Lois . . . "

She was helping a friend who was going through the same thing—breast cancer! *Thank You, Lord.* I told her about the armpit pain.

"Oh, Cindy's hurt too. I went over to help

her do her arm exercises. We put music on. She didn't get to start her radiation treatments right away because she couldn't get her arm up."

I made a mental note. *Do the arm exercises!* We talked a while longer and prayed together.

"I love you," I said.

"I love you too." she said, "I'll be praying."

"Good grief, just how many pray-ers are you going to get? If this keeps up we'll send for Doubt. . . . He's always a pro."

By the time Sunday came, I was eager to get out of my hovel a little. My spouse-nurse had been vigilant. My breast still did not hurt; my armpit still did. But the tube was draining less.

"I'll be really quiet. I won't overdo it. I'll just be sitting," I pleaded. Robert finally relented.

During a time of sharing in Sunday school several people praised God for my recovery and His faithfulness. Cheryl, our pastor's wife said, "I went over to see Lois and to cheer her up a little." She started to cry. "But instead she encouraged me."

Then I started to cry, because I was overcome with thankfulness to God. His word to me was "Stand ye *still*, and see the salvation of the LORD with you" (2 Chronicles 20:17b, KJV). Jehoshaphat and me. God was already proving His Word. It wasn't me. I'm a chicken when it comes to suffering.

*   *   *

I waited until I was forty-two to get my ears pierced! When Robert came home from work, I was lying on the couch.

"You're pale as a sheet! What happened?" he asked.

"I got my ears pierced."

"Did it hurt?"

"No," I cried. "It just seemed like it would!" For two weeks my nurse-friend Sharon had to do the alcohol cleansing. I couldn't bring myself to touch my ears!

*   *   *

I knew God was working a miracle in my life, turning a wimp into a vessel of honor for His glory. Church was wonderful but I was ever so glad to get back to my hovel and crawl into bed.

Later that afternoon, after I had a long nap, Carol came over. She sat in a chair at the end of the bed. Her directness was a quality I admired. "How are you staying so up?" she asked. She had gone through a very difficult surgery a few months earlier. It had been hard on her.

"Well, it must be because I'm so healthy. Remember that's what Dr. Fina said at my physical, at least before he found all this out." I knew

she didn't want to hear any pat spiritual answer. "And my Grandma Lennemann had a
breast removed in l935. It wasn't malignant, but
Grandma didn't have a breast. We all knew it.
She was still our wonderful Grandma. So why
can't I still be wonderful?" I joked.

I went on, "I just feel good. I feel really really
go—"

"No, that's not what I mean," she interrupted. "How do you stay so, so . . . so *up*? So
up spiritually?"

"Do you think I'm just stupid? Naive?" I
countered. "That I don't know this is cancer?
That I haven't grasped the seriousness of this?"

"That's what I'm beginning to think," she
said.

My innermost soul and thoughts went
through a quick personal exam. "I just have no
fear. I trust God. I believe His Word. Hundreds
of people are praying. Should we not see the
results of those prayers if God is who He says
He is?" I didn't quit there. I still had the floor
(well, the bed)!

"Second, what is the worst possible ending
to this? I could die, right? What happens
then? I go to heaven with God! That's not
bad. Third, another scenario, lots of chemo,
lots of pain? That could happen tomorrow.
God says take no thought about tomorrow,
today has enough trouble in itself, or something like that. Therefore I'm trusting Him for
that also."

She was starting to understand I thought.

"And I'm loving the history of Jehoshaphat in Second Chronicles 19 and 20. One verse says, 'Our eyes are on the Lord,' and this is where I want to be. You should read it."

I went on to tell her that I did not feel a glow or feel on some spiritual cloud. I just felt this quiet confidence in God. I also shared about having to deal with sins in my life, which was a relief.

After she left, I recorded the conversation in my journal. Another "Thank You, dear heavenly Father" went at the bottom of the page. After that I made a note, Psalm 27:4-6, KJV. Here is what that passage says:

> One *thing* have I desired of the LORD, that will I seek after; that I may dwell in the house of the LORD all the days of my life, to behold the beauty of the LORD, and to inquire in his temple. For in the time of trouble he shall hide me in his pavilion: in the secret of his tabernacle shall he hide me; he shall set me up upon a rock. And now shall mine head be lifted up above mine enemies round about me: therefore will I offer in his tabernacle sacrifices of joy; I will sing, yea, I will sing praises unto the LORD.

On Monday, Robert had to go to work. I stayed in bed. I wrote some thank-you notes.

And I tried to be as faithful as Robert in recording my day:

> Breakfast—peaches, cupcake
> little drainage
>
> Lunch—leftover casserole
>
> tube drained all guck and bloody stuff into bottle/clear liquid is running again/changed bandage myself

I kept my journal daily.

February 11:

Painted my fingernails (put fake ones on right hand). Going to speak at Sweetheart Banquet tonight, asked them to bring a stool. Later: I think I was more physically ready than I was emotionally. Afterthoughts plagued me all night long—I should've said this, should've said that. Couldn't sleep, maybe too much coffee!
> Don't forget: 2/12:
> Dr. Brown - 2:30 p.m.

"God is my Rock and my Fortress! Whom shall I fear?" *The doctor!!*

. . . the doctor taking the tape off under my arm. What if he takes that tube out?

"Greater is He that is in me than He that is in the world!" . . . at least it will get washed!

Robert went to work. I did some household chores. Then when he came home, we got the car loaded for our trip to Billings.

Sitting in the waiting room two hours later, we both thought of all that had transpired in two weeks.

"How are you doing?" I asked Robert. He looked older today, tired too.

"I'll be OK when you're OK. I just wish this was over."

I knew "this" referred to the test results. I had called Carewise, our company's health assistance program, and talked to the nurse. She had told me that the type of malignant tumor was a key factor in my prognosis. An estrogen-positive tumor was good news.

Robert had been talking to people also. He had some calls from spouses of breast cancer victims. "We've got to pray it's estrogen positive," he had told me earlier in the week.

Nurse Lisa, a ray of sunshine, called us back to the little room. "Dr. Brown will be with you in a few minutes."

"Hi folks," said Dr. Brown.

I stared at his name tag. I was determined this visit to get his first name. It filled the entire tag: Dr. Dennistoun Brown.

"I got the pathology report back," he said.

"And . . . ?" said Robert, who can be quite impatient when matters matter.

"The tumor was estrogen-progesterone positive . . ."

"Praise the Lord!" and that was from Robert, not me! I wasn't sure I understood all this yet.

"However . . ." (I thought later that Dr. Brown figured while we were celebrating such positive news, it would be a good time to toss in the down side.)

"However, there had been metastasis; the cancer had spread to one of the fifteen axillary lymph nodes I removed."

My ear picked up one word—"spread."

"Now tell me in English, just what does this mean?" I said from my perch on the exam table, wearing a blue paper gown—tied in front.

"It means this tumor was aggressive. I looked over your last year's mammogram. Usually you can see a shadow or indication of a tumor of this size when you look back. I could not see anything. Therefore this was aggressive. The tumor was 1.6 by 2.1 centimeters in size." He had me lie down on the table.

"The incision looks good. I tried to get it as low as possible."

"I certainly hope so," I countered. "I'd hate to have to throw away all my strapless evening gowns!"

He just smiled. I glanced at Robert. He was awfully quiet and very pale.

"Now what do we do?" I asked.

"You made the appointment with Dr. Lamm?" he asked.

I nodded. "I have an appointment on the 19th."

"I want you to see an oncologist also. You can make that appointment at the desk. Now let's see that left axillar."

"You mean my armpit? I'm scared about this. You know this is what hurts. My breast doesn't hurt, this hurts." I kept blabbing because I always do that when I'm nervous or scared. I was nervous and scared.

"Has it been draining much?"

"You have to ask Robert all the technical questions. He's charted it all. Here, I have a copy in my notebook." I gave Dr. Brown the meticulous notes Robert had made.

Dr. Brown looked them over. "I can remove it."

Pinching my thumbnail into my index finger on my right hand has always been my pain plan. If I pinch as hard as I can, it hurts enough to keep my mind off shots or blood tests, etc. In my head, I sang.

"Yuck!" How they had that much tube in my armpit, I'll never know. But it was out. Now Robert was relieved of irrigation duty.

Dr. Brown again went over the risks of lymphedema. Because of the lymph nodes being removed, infections could be a problem. The swelling of my arm would be reason for alarm.

He answered our questions, including a discussion of tamoxifen.

"Since your estrogen and progesterone receptors were positive, you are a good candidate for tamoxifen," Dr. Brown said. "Tamoxifen is an estrogen-blocking drug for long term use. But see what the oncologist has to say. It's not an option for everyone."

He got up and shook Robert's hand. Patting me on the shoulder, he said with a smile, "I'll see you in a month."

By random selection, Dr. Roger Santala was chosen to enter our lives as my oncologist. The process was simple—he had an opening on the 19th.

Robert looked decidedly better. "We can do it. And we've got a lot to thank God for."

He bowed his head and did just that. Out loud. The two of us—and God—in the little beige exam room with cotton swabs and tongue depressors. Thank God for every blessing.

    With Jehoshaphat . . .

    . . . we have no might against this great company that cometh against us; neither know we what to do: but our eyes *are* upon thee.
                    2 Chronicles 20:12 (KJV)

Chapter 8

File That Under "C" for Cancer

Like our expectations for the annual State of the Union and the State of the State speeches, I had assumptions about my future:

(drum roll please) . . .

The State of the Future
for Lois Olmstead
February 12, 1992

1. Cancer cells would be lurking in my body.

2. Chemotherapy would make me throwing-up sick.

3. I would lose my hair.

4. My husband would suffer greatly through this.

5. My folks would suffer greatly through this.

6. My family and friends would feel bad because of me.

7. I would be in the hospital.

8. I would be weaker and sicker than ever before in my life.

9. I would more than likely be dying.

10. God would be my strength whatever happened; I would trust Him.

Later, I realized that I was right about some of the assumptions and dead wrong about others. I didn't know much truth about cancer.

I knew about cancer only through people I had seen or heard about going through chemotherapy and what I had read or seen on television. The closest encounters that I had with cancer—besides the annual pap test, mammogram and the Cancer Drive—were with friends. Pat Hofeldt and Kitty Berube were friends. Both of them died of cancer. The experiences of these two friends were often in my mind. There were positive recollections also. Connie, Pat Nickel and Cheryl had breast cancer, and they were still alive. Annette DeLattre told me her mother had breast cancer thirty years ago. Her mom is still alive. And there were many famous people who had gone public as breast cancer survivors. Along with the ever-presence of my Savior and the faith of my husband, my friends helped me to have an optimistic view of life.

One of these friends was John Williams, a co-worker and neighbor. Enthusiastic, goodlooking, athletic, family oriented, kind and giving, John was involved in community activities and at the top of his field at work in Colstrip. A nagging, lower-leg ache threatened his daily running around the lake behind our houses. Several weeks, varied opinions and many tests later, the pain was diagnosed as a rare form of cancer, malignant schwannoma. Our community was shocked. No one as healthy and athletic as John could get cancer! But he did. He had chemotherapy, surgery and radiation. His wife Sandy, a nurse, was constant in her care and support as was the rest of his family.

John was going through aggressive chemo when I visited him in the hospital. He was pale. He was thin. I remember going over everything bad that had happened to Robert and me. I wanted him to know the sufficiency of God in all struggles. What a cheerful visit that must have been for John!

He impressed me with his decision to "fight with all I have; I am going to meet this disease head-on. I'm going to learn as much as I can going through this experience."

When John's daughter Sue graduated with our son Kevin in 1984 and John walked into the gymnasium with cap and cane, I cried. What a tragedy!

Yet John recovered! He jogs! He works! He treasures his grandchildren! He golfs—obsessively—and he checks in regularly with his doctors. He is *alive!* He was a role model for me. He was a silencer of those dark, whispering little arrows from my enemy.

"Cancer . . . pain . . . death."

I went back to work on February 13, ten days after surgery. In the morning I prayed that God would smooth the path ahead. I prayed that He would make me flexible to whatever happened. I wore a new bright-pink blouse with a blue skirt. Everyone was so kind. They were glad I was back. I put a piece of tape breast-high on the wall in the storage room. It took every ounce of my minuscule self-will, courage and discipline to raise my left arm and touch that tape with my hand. Every hour on the hour I went back to the storage room and painfully placed my hand on the tape and counted to ten. Co-workers reminded and encouraged me. I kept up the regimen faithfully every day, methodically raising the tape an inch at a time.

Karen's words inspired me: "Cindy couldn't start her radiation treatments because she couldn't get her arm raised." Sometimes I wondered if I even wanted to get my arm raised for radiation!

However, I was amazed at how quickly my arm was healing. It didn't seem to leak too much from the arm hole either. I did some errands downtown at lunch. I went home from work each night dog-tired. I went straight to the bed in my hovel. People brought supper almost every night. I would nap awhile. Then Robert would sit by my bed. We would eat supper together. Carol often joined us. We would pray, and I would go to sleep. Sometimes I would sleep through the night. Other nights were filled with tossing and turning.

The caring of people overwhelmed me. I recorded each day in my journal:

> 2/13 - Had more "givens" for supper. Pastor Mike came over. Called Lisa to say I wouldn't be at Bible study. My heart wanted to go but not my body. Carol came over with a funny card—I think it is the sixth one she has given me! After a little visit, decided to go with her to Bible study. Couldn't stand to miss it—went in robe—was great study. Psalm 73 is sure good in *Living Bible*. Robert came after me at 9 p.m. (his curfew)—changed bandages, to bed.

Our beliefs are a product of a lifetime of bits and pieces of information catalogued under various headings in our brain's file cabinet. This was so true with cancer and radiation therapy. Opinions had been formed, not necessarily factual. My brain file on radiation was not very full. But there were brain files nevertheless. Small scraps in my file looked something like this:

- My friend Isabel had gone through radiation. "It scares me to death. That big machine. No privacy. I wonder if it works?" she asked me.
- Some studies say radiation causes cancer, according to miscellaneous newspaper clippings, TV specials and news reports.
- My friend John went for radiation treatments. He lost all his hair, but he's doing great now, four years later. And his hair is back too.

That's about all I knew. But I also knew that things change. So I read the brochures on radiation therapy given to me at the hospital. They said the treatments would take around thirty minutes.

"Do you know where that little red Walkman tape player is?" I asked Robert.

"Yes, it's downstairs on the storage shelves. Why?"

"Well, I want to play tapes while I'm getting radiated. You know I could take some praise tapes and hymns and play them while they are zapping me."

"Lois," he said, "you would fry the tapes."

"Oh."

I called our neighbors John and Sandy Williams. "Could you guys come over this evening? I need to ask you about 200 million questions."

"We'd be glad to," said Sandy. "We were planning on coming over this weekend anyway."

It was good to see an older member of the club I had just been initiated into. "Older" as in survivor. "Club" as in Cancer Club. He was a member of the Malignant Schwannoma Chapter; I was a member of the Breast Cancer Chapter.

"I have to tell you what an inspiration you have been to me these last two weeks," I said to John. "I just keep thinking, John went through all this and he's still living!"

John laughed. "I know just what you mean. Now it seems so long ago."

"First thing I want to know . . . How was the driving back and forth every day to Billings?" The Northern Rockies Cancer Center is located in Billings. Patients living outside of Billings have several options. Staying with family or friends or in motels with special rates for medical patients are the most popular choices.

"We went in the morning," replied John. "I have the most energy in the morning. I felt my best time should be devoted to curing my cancer. When we got back to Colstrip, Sandy drove me right to the high school. I swam for a half hour, then I went home, showered and went to work."

"I hadn't thought about that. I'm a morning person too."

Robert liked the morning idea. "Then I wouldn't have to worry about you driving home in the dark and hitting a deer."

"OK, we'll try for mornings," I said. "Then I'll just work in the afternoons."

"Did you think driving every day was a pain?" I asked.

"Not at all," they both said at once.

"It was one of the best times for the two of us," Sandy said. "We talked more and communicated feelings better than any other time in our marriage."

John looked at Sandy and laughed. "We almost need to do it again!"

"Now next question. How long do you really get zapped? I told Robert I wanted to play my praise tapes, and he said I would fry them."

John was smiling again. "No, you don't want your tapes, Lois. You won't have time. The actual radiation isn't much longer than an X-ray. Of course, it depends on your particular treatment."

"Well, I'll know that tomorrow. I start regular treatments on Friday and chemotherapy the same day."

"That soon?" John asked. "I started chemotherapy before my surgery. That's when I lost all my hair. It was falling out all over my pillow. I finally just called the nurse. I was in the hospital waiting for the surgery, and I just told her to give me a buzz. I hated just waiting for it all to fall out."

"Will you lose your hair?" asked Sandy.

I reached up to touch my hair. "My oncologist said that one-third of the women on the program I'm on do lose all their hair, one-third don't and one-third lose some."

"We just have to wait and see," interjected Robert. "We'll cross that bridge when we get to it."

Once again, I was comforted by his "we." *Thank You, Lord!* I opened the gifts they brought. Sandy gave me a stuffed nurse-bear with its left arm in a sling. Sandy is an RN and knew what my left arm felt like. John gave me a gift of an old man whittled out of wood.

"Is this hoping we'll both grow old?" I joked.

"Just put it in your car. Take it with you on your trips."

Robert showed them to the door. I was busy rearranging my brain file cabinet. Things were changing in there already. I needed to get my notebook so we could draw up a schedule.

Chapter 9

Welcome to the Rad Club

Our appointment with Dr. Frank Lamm, my radiation doctor, was scheduled for 8 a.m., February 19 at the Northern Rockies Cancer Center in Billings. The Northern Rockies Cancer Center. The *Cancer* Center. The building had a gold roof and bold architectural lines—ultra-modern with a high arched canopy over the driveway.

A medical transit van was parked under the canopy. The driver was unloading a patient in a wheelchair. We walked in the door with a few butterflies trying to get a flight pattern established in our stomachs. I had asked our church family to pray that I would be able to raise my left arm over my head for this appointment, which was critical to the getting-set-up process. So my main concern was an athletic endeavor, and I don't have an athletic bone in my body.

*   *   *

Memories of exercise and physical education classes in high school and college still haunt my nightmares. Getting married and having three boys didn't help.

"Why doesn't Mom want to get in the water, Dad?" they'd holler from the lakeshore.

He couldn't say, "Because she's afraid you'll tip her air mattress over!" That would make me sound like a chicken, and, where boys are concerned, that's the same as throwing a red flag in front of a raging bull. So God and a master-of-intimidation instructor taught me to swim at the YMCA.

Yet that wasn't enough for my family. Robert and the boys gave me a bike for my birthday. It was yellow and had a basket covered with plastic daisies on it. They knew I would love it. Of course, I said I did.

We rode horses on the ranch where I grew up. Gravel roads just weren't conducive to bikes. So I had to learn to herd this bike down the street without reins, hoping all the kids wouldn't be laughing at me at the ripe old age of twenty-nine. I practiced and practiced riding that bright yellow bike.

Several days later I got into a baking spree. Those are few and far between in my kitchen. I was ready to bake a cake: one box of cake mix, one-half cup water, two eggs.

But I was out of eggs. *I know what I'll do*, I thought. *I'll just bike over to the 7-Eleven and get the eggs.* I put on the new bright-pink jogging suit I had bought so I could look athletic. Then out the door I went and hopped on my bike for the three-block ride.

I told everyone in the store that I had biked over to purchase my eggs. I think they already knew, because it took me five minutes to get my bike leaned up against the store like I had seen the kids do. Also I was panting and gulping for air.

I paid for the eggs and put them in the daisy-covered basket. Then I breathed a prayer and headed for home.

The three-block ride went well. I was feeling quite confident. I had never done curbs before. The curb by our driveway was just a small one, so I braced myself and pointed my bike straight up the driveway.

When I hit the curb, the eggs flew out of the basket. The blue carton of one dozen grade AA eggs landed on the driveway in front of my bike. I rode straight over the carton . . . breaking every single egg.

Then I had to get the car out of the garage (so I could go to a different grocery store) and buy more eggs. I also had to change clothes because I didn't feel very athletic anymore.

*   *   *

Now you understand, I don't have an athletic bone in my body . . . but God loves me anyway. The very fact that I had done the arm exercises was a miracle. I had been working on the exercises since I had been dismissed from the hospital. I gritted my teeth and prayed *Help, Lord* (that was becoming a regular prayer), as I walked my fingers up the wall to touch the tape.

I could hardly believe it. That arm, which I was sure would never wave at a friend or raise in praise to God again, was loosening up. Higher and higher. *Thank You, God, one more time. Thank You, God.*

So there we were at the Northern Rockies Cancer Center. Our first appointment. The first of many. But I wasn't thinking about that. I wasn't thinking about the setup procedure or the awesomeness of the high-tech equipment. As Robert and I walked through the door I was thinking about the Olympics.

I was so proud of how high God had enabled me to raise my arm that I couldn't wait to show the doctor. I was becoming athletic, even with cancer.

The atrium at the Northern Rockies Cancer Center was made possible by a donation from Alberta Bair, a local philanthropist, along with many others. God bless them. It is beautiful and comfortable.

"Robert! There are ducks!" I squealed. In the middle of the atrium were eight ducks swimming under a little bridge. I felt one of those goose bump-buzzes flow over me. *Praise God! Thank You, God!*

* * *

In Colstrip some kids call me the duck lady. Seeking a new adventure a few years ago, I decided to get baby ducks. We lived on the edge of Castle Rock Lake, so it seemed to be a great idea.

I ordered the ducks from Forsyth Seed Company and then went home to enlist my husband's engineering expertise in building their home. We used a borrowed rabbit hutch for their house. It took fifty feet of chicken wire to totally enclose the pen. I bought waterers and feeders and even added a covered patio.

They arrived at the post office, peeping through the holes in a little box. There were twenty-two fuzzy brown ducks. Their pen seemed awfully big when I put them in. Ducks stick together. I mean really together. Wherever they go, it's in a pack. The little fuzzy pack runs to the water—together. Then they run to the food—together. If one lies down, they all lie down. When one gets up, they all get up. It's like one moves and the others say, "That's a good idea!"

Being the ducks' stepmom became quite time consuming. They were always out of water or food, and when it rained the pen required constant cleaning. I hadn't thought about getting up at 6 o'clock to slosh out in the rain to feed my adventure or stumbling down to the darkened lake at night to get another pail of water.

Soon I was ready to turn them out on the lake. I hoped that they automatically knew how to swim or it would be back to the YMCA for us all. They swam.

A few days later I went down to feed them. They were swimming in the lake. They came when I called and ate with gusto. Then they ran for their new bigger-than-olympic-size swimming pool.

I wasn't the only one attached to these little creatures. Adults and children from our community came to feed them. Fishermen on the lake tried to ignore them. I wrote about them in my newspaper column.

Once we had to cut a fish hook out of Willard's leg. He barely survived. I had to give him shots of antibiotics for four days. Throughout the next few months, I wasn't only the ducks' mom but their vet as well. Picking up lost fish hooks became a common malady. I got quite handy as Dr. Duck Lady.

Naturally one thing led to another. Pretty soon I was buying Monte Dolack duck prints. I bought duck-bordered wallpaper for my office in our home. Then some ceramic ducks. Then a duck quilt, duck curtains . . .

Last night someone stopped by our house. He said, "I wasn't sure which house you lived in, but when I saw the duck curtains in the window, I knew this must be the one."

* * *

So you can imagine how I felt walking into the Cancer Center.

There were ducks!

There were ducks!

God, I'm just overwhelmed. I know these people don't even know who Lois Olmstead is yet and thinking that You had them put those ducks there just for me seems more than impossible.

Of course, You are always doing "impossible" miracles. So I'm just going to say, *"Thank You, God." This is proof to me that You will be here in this place, the Cancer Center, with me.*

We told the receptionist who we were. We were Lois Olmstead.

I was so thankful that God and Robert were with me each step of the way. I knew that not everyone understands that God wants and desires to be their friend and companion. God says in His Word, "I will lead the blind [and cancer people] by ways they have not known, along unfamiliar paths I will guide them; I will turn the darkness into light before them and make the rough places smooth. These are the things I will do; I will not forsake them" (Isaiah 42:16, NIV).

I also knew that not everyone had a loving spouse or friend to go with them. I breathed a "Thank You, Lord" prayer for His presence. And Robert's.

At 8 a.m. an attractive woman with friendly eyes, beautiful gray hair and a smile on her face called my name. We went together, the three of us. God, Robert and me.

The nurse wore a white uniform. She had a blue notebook in her hand with "Lois Olmstead" on a red tag across the end of it. I smiled and got another one of those goose bump-buzzes.

Lord, I just can't believe this. I mean, yes, I do believe it. You really do want me to feel at home here.

Besides ducks, my other addiction is notebooks. I have big notebooks and little notebooks. I have pink ones, flowered ones, ones with pockets, some with dividers, some for single purposes. I carry a notebook instead of a purse.

Here at the Cancer Center they had notebooks too!

As we followed this nurse through the double doors, I started singing in my head. Me and Jehoshaphat, *Count your many blessings, name them one by one. Count your many blessings, see what God hath done.*

The nurse's name was Pauline. She chatted with us as she led us down the hall and into a small room. We sat down in the patient chairs.

My time at the Northern Rockies Cancer Center had come. Reality checked in.

"Curtain call! Curtain call!"
"Did we forget to mention a few things when we gave you our sales pitch? Oh, well, you'll find out. Surgery is the regular stuff. This is our arena now. Cancer. Radiation. Chemotherapy. You're on stage, but we're the stars."

Pauline opened the blue Lois-notebook and checked the information there. We were who the book said we were. We were where we were supposed to be at the time the book said.

"We have a video about radiation therapy," she said. "It will answer a lot of questions about the equipment and treatment." She put the film in and turned up the volume. "After you watch the video, I'll answer any questions about it that you might have."

Robert grabbed my hand. We watched the ten-minute film. We saw pictures of the equipment. We watched the technicians do their thing. The film showed the treatment procedure I would soon experience. New words were entered into my mind-dictionary. I got a new vocabulary, a cancer vocabulary. The film ended. No one served popcorn.

Nurse Pauline came back. I liked her because she was upbeat. She didn't seem to think the

Cancer Treatment play, act one, had to be a tragedy. I was encouraged by her attitude.

After a few explanations, she led us down
the hall to an exam room. We walked by a hospital patient on a stretcher waiting for her turn
for treatment. The ambulance attendant stood
by her side.

Then we passed the inner waiting room.
When I became a bona fide member, I found
out this was an exclusive club room. Out in the
atrium there were spouses and friends plus for-
mer patients waiting for their checkups. But in
this little vestibule sat patients waiting for their
turns at radiation. I named this the Rad Club. I
thought about printing up a sign:

Rad Club

—Members and Invited Guests Only—

Soon I learned how successful the cancer re-
cruiting business was. This particular treatment
center began fifteen years ago and treats up to
sixty patients on some days. The staff fre-
quently comes in early and works late to ac-
commodate the schedules of so many patients.
I checked out these patients as I walked by the
Rad Club waiting area—they sure looked like
regular people to me.

————————

*"We told you we had an excellent
random selection process, didn't we? Our
selection process crosses all walks of life. All*

*ages. All types of people. And just think, we
found you too. You didn't even have to
audition."*

"Here we are," said nurse Pauline. "Dr. Lamm will be right with you."

"I can't remember what he looks like, can you?" I asked Robert. We were sitting side by side in the mauve upholstered patient chairs.

He was getting that pale I-wish-this-wasn't-happening-to-you look again.

I didn't wait for his answer. "I was still out there in woo-woo land when he came to the hospital. I remember he was there. He told me he had looked at my reports. And he said we'd see him later. That's about all I can remember about him."

I raised my left arm up over my head. I just had to make sure it still performed on cue. I put it back down on my lap.

"Hello, I'm Dr. Lamm," the doctor announced as he came into the room. He shook hands with Robert. He sat down in the doctor chair. And then he looked at me. "How are you doing? You were still a little groggy when I met you in the hospital."

He remembered. And he really did seem to care. *Dear Lord*, I thought, *is this another blessing You have for me?*

Dr. Lamm opened the blue Lois-notebook. "I have several things to go over with you." He brought out a form with lots of blank lines. "This is a required procedure to inform you of some of the effects of radiation therapy."

He went over the possible side effects of my treatment. We asked questions. He patiently answered each one. We were sliding right into act one, scene one, *Cancer Treatment*. It was apparent that Dr. Lamm was one of the main actors in this play. He was my radiation oncologist. He was the one who would determine the radiation treatment and follow-up for my particular cancer.

I think I might even be the main character in this play, I thought. Me, who had never even made it into a high school play.

"That's just what we had in mind. Now you're getting the picture."

Dr. Lamm left the room to get another report. He left the blue Lois-notebook on the doctor desk.

I looked at Robert and said, "What would you do if the doctor left your chart in your exam room?"

"Why?"

"Because I'm me, and me wants to look in there," I said as I reached for it. I read the report on my tumor. There were a few words I didn't know the meaning of or even how to pronounce. It looked like they had told me everything in the report. There were no new surprises or information that the doctors had not shared with me. That took care of the maybe-they-aren't-telling-me-everything worry. *Thank You, Lord.* (Is it OK to thank God for snooping?) The report also had a big empty chart in it, with lots of spaces for the days ahead.

"Looks good to me, the notebook expert," I sheepishly told Robert as I put it back in its exact spot. "I think it's OK to look at your records," I said to eradicate my guilt. "This is the '90s, you know."

Dr. Lamm returned. "Now the next question. How is your arm?"

"I thought you'd never ask," I said. I went to the wall and walked my arm well up over my head. I almost expected to hear the "Star Spangled Banner" and see an American flag unfurled in the room.

"That's really good! Excellent!" said Dr. Lamm.

Now I knew that I liked this doctor. He recognized my great athletic endeavor. "I had people in my church praying for my arm," I said.

"That means we can get started right away."

"Like how right away?" I asked.

"Right now," he said. "The simulation is the next step. The nurse will show you to the room."

I whispered to Robert, "I think right now I wish I hadn't been so ambitious. Then I could put this off . . . no, I don't. Let's get this show on the road."

"Curtain call! Curtain call! Lois Olmstead, Dr. Lamm, technical staff . . . oh yes, bring the husband too."

I had done my homework. I had read every bulletin and brochure I had been given in the hospital. I knew that the simulation involved a machine which aided doctors in planning the treatment for each individual need. They use it to outline the treatment area and all the angles and distances for the linear accelerator.

The real "radiator" is the linear accelerator, which would direct a precisely-defined beam of radiation at my cancer site to destroy any cancer cells that might be left after surgery. The simulation was used to set up a program especially designed for me—personalized and unique.

I thought the aqua-blue gown should have a designer label. But when I put on the gown, I knew this place had its act together. The gown fastened in the front. Maybe the label came later.

The room was right out of *Star Trek*. Robert was fascinated by all the equipment and so was I. Having an engineer for a husband, I had toured control rooms in electric generating plants and hydroelectric plants throughout the West. *Thank You, Lord. You even prepared me for all of the complicated equipment.*

What happened next was the beginning of friendships with some of the most caring, empathetic, sincere people I have ever met—the Cancer Center staff. The technician introduced herself. She explained again what they would be doing. She told me my part would be to lie very still on the table. I really did feel like an actress in a play.

ACT Two: Introduction to Radiation Therapy

Scene One:

(Dr. Lamm directs a complex program with the aid of X-rays, computers, monitors and the simulator to set up the best possible angles for radiation with the least possible risks to the patient's surrounding tissue.)

Also starring: two technicians, one husband and the patient.

ACTION!

"Now we want you to lie back on this bag. It will feel slightly warm," said the technician-nurse. "I'll help you as you lie back into it slowly."

I did as instructed. I was lying with my upper body cradled in a black garbage bag filled with goo.

"We're making your cradle," the tech said. "This is like liquid styrofoam. It hardens very quickly. We need to have you put your arm up over your head. Lay your other hand on your waist. Lois, you are going to have to lie still for a very long time."

The brochure from the U.S. Department of Health and Human Services had explained this procedure:

> In a process called simulation (a major step in planning your treatment), you will be asked to lie very still on a table while a technologist uses a special machine to X-ray the cancer and locate your treatment port. This is the exact place on your body where the high-energy rays will be aimed. Simulations may take about two hours. (Publication no. 88-2227)

Dr. Lamm was at my side. Another technician was on my right. Robert was in the guest chair a few feet away. *This is some show*, I thought. *I haven't had so much high-tech personalized attention in my whole life!*

My next honest-to-goodness prayer was not very spiritual, but it came straight from my heart:

Dear Lord, I thank You that my cancer is on the top. I just don't think my vanity could handle a styrofoam mold of my bottom! I didn't catch His reply.

My arm! Jehoshaphat, I think the enemy is here. I can see them lining up on the horizon. The Moabites are ready to begin slinging their arrows. Does my arm have to stay over my head forever?

If I could barely take getting my ears pierced, and that didn't even really hurt, how am I going to handle this? This hurts! So, Jehoshaphat, here we go.

> And when he [Jehoshaphat] had consulted with the people, he appointed singers unto the LORD, and that should praise the beauty of holiness, as they went out before the army, and to say, Praise the LORD; for his mercy endureth for ever. And when they began to sing and to praise, the LORD set ambushments against . . . Ammon, Moab, and mount Seir, . . . and they were smitten. (2 Chronicles 20:21-22, KJV)

And that was the beginning. The beginning of my singing before the Lord when my body was under siege. The beginning of lying still and letting invisible rays that I could not see, hear or feel work in my body. My part was just to praise my Lord and let Him and His caregivers do their job.

———————

"The cameras are rolling. Let's just see if your faith is real . . . or something you Christians just like to talk about. We're

going to give you a taste of the real action.
By the way, we don't use stuntmen.
You are on—now."

Praise God from whom all blessings flow . . .
Praise Him all creatures here below . . .
hmm hmmm hmmmm . . .
Father, Son and Holy Ghost. Amen.

Jesus giveth us the victory,
He who overcame on Calvary . . .
hmm . . . hmm . . . hmmm . . .
Jesus giveth us the victory. . .

Onward Christian soldiers marching on to war,
with the cross of Jesus going on before.
Forward into battle with our banner raised.
On before the . . . hmmm, hmm, hmmm . . .

Yes, you're right. There's a battle raging. Now I feel it. Someone or something is trying to rob me of my concentration. I can't think straight. Is it the radiation already? My mind feels under siege.

I could not pull the words of songs from my memory. Songs I had sung for years and had known every word by heart.

For a moment it was frightening. *Lord, how can I sing praise songs to You in the midst of battle if I can't remember the words?*

Then there was that still, small voice that

speaks to us who are children of the King. He calmed my feeling of near panic. Words were written in my mind at that precise moment by the Holy Spirit.

Not the words of the songs I was trying to sing in my head. These words:

"Lois, just praise Me.
Praise Me with your words.
Parts of songs,
Parts of Scripture,
just praise Me."

It was as clear as if God had sent me a telegram. From then on, I just praised Him. With songs . . . I couldn't always remember all the lines. With Scripture . . . and I couldn't always remember all the words. But I praised Him with my whole being whenever I was "under the gun."

Not out loud, of course. I'm a lousy singer. I can sing really well when I'm standing by someone else who sings really well—like in choir at church. But alone? No thank you. Not at all.

For the next several weeks I did a lot of singing during radiation. Quiet singing. But it sure was loud in my head, because I was praising God with my whole heart. Jehoshaphat and me.

"For we have no might against this great company that cometh against us; neither know we what to do: but our eyes are upon thee" (2 Chronicles 20:12, KJV).

"Well, maybe we lost a little ground there with our confusion maneuver, but we'll try the pain tactic—that's a sure-fire approach. Write it into the script."

My arm was still over my head. Dr. Lamm and the technicians were in and out of the room as they did different calculations and measurements. Every now and then they would take an X-ray. Then Robert had to leave the room.

The simulator was changed at times to different angles. As numbers flashed on a computer screen over in the corner, I felt in awe. All of this technology was being focused on me alone. I could tell that Dr. Lamm had a setup in his mind for my particular cancer. And he wasn't going to settle for "close." He wanted it perfect to the millimeter, or however you gauge radiation.

"Blessed is the man that walketh not in the counsel of the ungodly, nor standeth in the way of sinners, nor sitteth in the seat of the scornful. But his delight is in the law of the LORD, *and in his law doth he meditate day and night"* (Psalm 1:1-2, KJV).

There! I said one all the way through. I don't know if I got all the standing and sitting right. But it was close. I just kept singing songs and quoting verses while this team of specialists worked around me.

Robert stopped every time he passed on his way to the shielded room when they did an X-ray and said, "How are you doing?" or whispered, "I love you."

The technicians and Dr. Lamm were drawing marks on my left breast, up my neck to my lymph nodes there and under my arm. Once in a while they looked in my eyes and said, "Are you doing all right?" or "It won't be much longer."

"I'm fine," I replied. And to my surprise I was fine. I know I shouldn't have been surprised. My prayer supporters—people who committed themselves to pray for me—were praying for me as I was in the arena. I had specifically asked them to pray that I would be able to hold my arm up as long as necessary.

"Well, we didn't count on reinforcements. We'll up that pain level just a little. Act three, scene two, take six . . . Action!"

It did hurt. But not unbearably. My foot went to sleep. That was a real distraction. *If I could move my foot a little.*

"Now Lois we want you to lie very still. We're taking another X-ray," said Jan, the technician.

Couldn't move. Had to lie still. *My foot hurts.*

Drats! Didn't tell anybody to pray for my feet! OK Jehoshaphat, "Mine eyes have seen the glory of the coming of the Lord. . . ." Does that qualify for a hymn?

"We're almost done," Dr. Lamm said. "How are you doing?"

"OK," I said. I was hanging on to a wisp of my bangs to keep my arm up in the right position. And I was OK. Yes, my arm hurt some. My foot hurt some. I was OK. Some of my songs and verses were reruns by now. But that was OK too. Each time I said them I remembered more lines.

Another interesting phenomenon of the simulation experience was this: I'm a pretty modest person. Yet in that room at some point in time, my modesty took a back seat to medical necessity. From that moment my body, in my mind, became sort of a medical laboratory specimen (speciwoman?). I didn't feel embarrassed or even shy or uncomfortable. My breast needed medical attention. It was just all a part of the battle plan. I thank God for changing me. How I appreciated the sensitivity of the medical team as I crossed this hurdle. (Besides, I still had my designer aqua-blue gown, you know, for "public" appearances and all.)

"That's it." Jan held my hand. "Now you can put your arm down."

"No, I don't think I can put my arm down," I said. I wasn't even sure I could let go of my hair. I had to take hold of my left arm with my right hand. Ever so slowly I lifted it down to my side. What relief! It was over.

It was over. The two-hour simulation that I had read about.

It was over. I smiled. Another bridge crossed. *Thank You, Lord.*

Now the next challenge: I had to get my body off the table. I couldn't get up.

"Now just take it easy," said Jan, the technician who now had my respect and admiration for her intelligence with this awesome equipment. "I'll help you up. Just take it slowly."

I made it! Robert was right by my side. I sat there awhile to get rid of the fuzzy feeling in my legs. I could begin to feel my feet again. I still had two of them. The left one didn't fall off after all.

"Now you'll have to be very careful with these marks we have on you," Dr. Lamm said. "Don't wash them off . . . or we'll have to do this all over again."

He couldn't have said anything to impress me more. I would wear an umbrella in the shower. No way was I going to wash off those marks. They had to stay until permanent ones could be tatooed in their place. I never desired a tattoo. But I would get six tiny-blue-dot tattoos to decorate me for the rest of my life.

"Maybe I could get them to do a little duck instead of a dot," I said to Robert. "At least I would have something to show for the pain."

"No," he said. "No ducks."

Dr. Lamm told us he would meet with a physicist and other technologists to make personalized lead blocks for me. These blocks would be designed from the information they had collected through the simulations and from the X-rays taken before and after my surgery to remove the malignant tumor. My very own personalized blocks would enable the radiation to be focused exactly on my cancer site, or "port" as the medical people call it. They also call it "the field."

I went from breast to port to field. Well, that's appropriate for my battle plan. Battles usually do take place on a battlefield. *Thank You, Lord. You knew this all along!*

Dr. Lamm asked if we had any more questions. "If not, we'll see you tomorrow night at 5:30." He had the blue Lois-notebook under his arm. "Plan on at least an hour as we get you set up on the linear accelerator. The first time usually takes a little longer. Then we'll start your treatments on Friday."

He smiled as he handed us back to nurse Pauline. I breathed another prayer. *Thank You, Lord, for a compassionate, smart doctor. Glad You picked him out. You're two for two!*

We walked down the hall. Different people were sitting in the Rad Club. Normal everyday people. One lady looked about my age. She had one of the aqua-blue gowns on over her jeans. I wondered if she had breast cancer too.

"That will be you tomorrow. A patient. Waiting to be zapped. Your membership card comes with the notebook. You have joined the club. You have a cancer label now. You're one of us."

"Lois, we'd like to get your picture. And then I'll show you our dressing rooms," Pauline said.

This must be my I.D. tag so I can join the club, I thought.

She showed us four dressing rooms. "Pick a number, one that will be easy for you to remember."

"I'll choose two." I was born in 1942. I hoped I could remember later why I was supposed to remember 1942.

She took a piece of masking tape and wrote Olmstead on it. She stuck it over a hook. "That will be where your gown is every day when you come in."

I glanced at the names on the other hooks. I recognized one. "Now your appointment for a CAT scan at the Deaconess Hospital is at 11:30 a.m. That's a half hour from now. Then we'll see you tomorrow night at 5:30."

I was glad I had just written "Medical Stuff" on my notebook page for today's schedule. Robert and I walked out through the atrium. I paused to talk to the ducks. "Guess we'll be getting acquainted. I'll be here often."

"Looks like duck heaven to me," Robert said. "There are no dogs or coyotes to get after them. No snow or ice in the winter. Plenty of water and food. 'Spose your ducks will wind up here?"

"Of course," I agreed. "I did, didn't I?"

We walked the block from the parking lot of the Northern Rockies Cancer Center to the Deaconess Hospital. We met my mom for coffee in the cafeteria. She had come from Livingston to be with us.

We had stepped into a new world, the world of cancer treatment. "One small step for . . ."

"Seeing is believing. You didn't think this play was going to run without some hands-on experience did you? Let's just call it doing some real life research. You're just getting started."

Radiation—Application

1. Do the exercises that your doctor tells you to do. Count any pain as a small step toward victory. If you do it inch by inch, you can persevere. These ideas will help:

   a. Ask people to pray for you.

   b. Sing praise songs.

    c. Have someone help you. (A friend of mine in Texas used this as her special ministry to a breast cancer patient. She went over to her house and coached her and prayed with her.)

    d. Say Bible verses.

    e. Remember me—if unathletic, pansy me can do it . . . so can you!

2. Remember to look for adventure. Learn as much as you can about your treatment. Ask questions. Watch for God's blessings as you walk your path.

3. If the equipment is frightening to you as you walk into the room, ask the technologist to explain its purpose. When you understand the process, it will be less frightening.

4. Be sure to take a friend with you. It helps to have them listening to all the information with you.

5. Always remember that God is with us as His children. He has promised to be with us—even in the Rad Room!

Bible References

One morning during my treatment when my blood count was very low, I was quarantined to my house. I got a call from our pastor. "Lois, there's a group of ladies gathered out here at the church praying just for you. I just thought you'd be encouraged to know that."

Oh, I was so touched and humbled and encouraged and uplifted. Later they dropped off notes of love and a list of verses they felt God had given them for me. I want to share those with you:

Lamentations 3:19-26 Acts 1:14
Galatians 6:2   Romans 15:30-33
1 Peter 3:12   Jeremiah 29:11-13
Psalm 41:3   Psalm 50:15

Chapter 10

Facing the Enemy in the Dark

At 11:30 a.m. I reported to the Deaconess Hospital for a CAT scan of my upper body. This was a base-line procedure. My mom, Robert and I went to the radiology department. A nurse told us to wait, so we sat down on the light blue chairs under an attractive floral print in an oak frame.

There were three women in the room. Two were in wheelchairs. One was without hair and very weak. She moaned softly. The other woman had red, splotchy bruises on her face and neck. The third woman was about my age. Her body was thin. She had a turban around her scalp and looked very weak. She sat across from us.

I tried to smile cheerily as I grabbed for Robert's hand. My mom looked like she could cry.

"Hey guys! Great to see you!" said Dennis Hully, a good friend who worked in this department. "Marcia told me about your news.

Sure does seem to be a lot of cancer." He shook his head. "Three of our friends are going through just what you are right now." He led me into the room where the CAT scan would be taken.

My most vivid memory is of pain. I had to raise my arm over my head yet keep it close enough to my body to allow the cylinder over my body. This was getting to be a regular routine. Maybe I was going to be eligible for an Olympic event. I grabbed for the same lock of hair I had clung to earlier in the day.

Then I let go of it quickly. *Good grief! No sense pulling it out ahead of time!*

After two hours of raised-arm positions at the Cancer Center, my muscles were in a knot. Tears came to my eyes. "Dennis, I just can't do it!"

"You're OK. You're doing fine. Just hold it right there. We'll be done soon."

Soon wasn't quick enough for me, but I managed to lie still. I started to sing in my head. *OK, Jehoshaphat, don't quit now. We've got to sing.* Through the "Battle Hymn of the Republic" and "Jesus Loves Me," I lay still.

"That hurt!" I told Robert as we left the hospital.

We grabbed a quick lunch. Then we went back to the Billings Clinic for our appointment with my oncologist. I was still learning how to say the word.

Later the oncology waiting room would become a favorite place for me. It was where I could meet other cancer-type people. I could see hope, courage, faith and inspiration in the faces, fighting faces.

Be forewarned. The first visit may not be so inspirational. This day I saw the enemy, cancer, at its finest. Old people, young people, women like me. Spouses like Robert. Fear, in frightening fury, flooded my soul. My future was sitting around me.

The Billings Clinic always has a jigsaw puzzle out on the coffee table in the oncology waiting room. Robert knelt beside the table, searching for a piece to fit the peaceful farm scene. I sat rigid in my chair.

A tall nurse in a white pants suit came into the room. She looked down at the chart, "Mrs. Olmstead?" I stood up and Robert was right behind me.

That was the last time I ever saw any staff look at a chart for my name. I don't know how they do it, but the clinic staff and those at the Cancer Center always know I am Lois. And they know all the other patients by name also. When your basic trust in your body has been destroyed by cancer, it means so much to have that personal touch of being recognized.

They led me to the scales. I had lost six pounds since my physical. Normally I would have been excited about that. We were shown into a small exam room, but not before I saw the three window rooms. These rooms had recliners, televisions, lots of magazines, some chairs—and a few people getting chemotherapy by injection. The windows made it possible for nurses to watch the patients.

The nurse took my medical history. Then before leaving she said, "You may put on the gown, and Dr. Santala will be with you shortly."

"So I wonder what this doctor will be like?" I said to Robert.

"I don't know, but we'll soon find out."

"I hope he's like the others have been, friendly, full of conversation and easy to talk with."

Dr. Santala flunked all of the above. He was tall, very confident, stern and distant. I didn't like him.

After this visit I conducted a survey. I asked all the cancer people I knew who their doctor was. No one said Dr. Santala except Lisa Olson's family—and Lisa had died. On my next visit to Dr. Brown I told him about my survey, "Just tell me the truth," I said. "Does he have any survivors?"

He roared! "Dr. Roger Santala is an excellent oncologist. You're in good hands . . . and *yes* he does have survivors!"

Later I learned that I was indeed in excellent hands. Roger is one of my favorite doctors now. He isn't stern and distant—he is friendly, brilliant, professional, and he does a great beaver imitation!

But this day I was not only disappointed, I was irritated. He wouldn't look me in the eye. He kept glancing at my watch. Granted, it is a wonderful watch. It was a gift from Robert at Christmas. The band is red. It has flags of different countries on the face—and the face moves instead of the hands. I covered the watch with my other hand.

Dr. Santala started with the same procedure as Dr. Lamm—the risks and side effects of chemotherapy! I thought, *Radiation and chemotherapy are conceivably poisons rather than the antidote!*

I need to confess that in the back of our minds, both Robert and I had assumed I would not be getting chemotherapy. A friend of ours had breast cancer fours years earlier. Her husband had called Robert right after he found out about my cancer. Her lump was similar in size to mine. Hers was estrogen receptor positive. She was on the new drug tamoxifen and would be taking the drug for the rest of her life.

"I could live with that," I told Robert when I heard. "Maybe that is God's healing drug."

That was not the drug of choice for my cancer. Dr. Santala said I would be on a CMF protocol. A protocol is a specific plan with set guidelines for the purpose of research or study. Dosages and frequency of administration of chemo drugs are rigidly set for a specific type of patient.

CMF is a combination of cyclophosphamide (more commonly called cytoxin) plus methotrexate plus fluorouracil. Dr. Santala told us I would be taking the cytoxin orally. The methotrexate and fluorouracil would be administered by injection.

"Now are you getting the picture? That will be you out there in the window chair."

An even bigger shock to us than not taking tamoxifen was that I would be doing chemotherapy and radiation at the same time. I had never heard of such a thing!

"See? You really are dying. That's why they are hitting all sides . . . if the side effects don't get you, we will!"

Side effect words were hitting my soul like arrows:

muscle or bone pain	nausea
shortness of breath	fever, chills
stomach pain	loss of appetite
hair loss	sores in mouth
tiredness	

"I really doubt you will lose all of your hair on this program," Dr. Santala said. "Many of my patients with hair as thick as yours do not."

Well, thanks for the ray of good news! I thought. *What's a little hair to throwing up, canker sores, muscle pain, fever and fatigue!* I was getting quite nasty. I wasn't singing anymore at all!

"We've got you now! So much for your Jehoshaphat victory song! And look at your husband—we wounded him too! He's green!"

Dr. Santala stood up. He shook Robert's hand and touched mine. I tried to dismiss his act of kindness. "I will schedule your first injection for Friday," he said.

"This Friday?" I stammered.

"Yes." He went out the door and closed it behind him.

"Well, we can do this," Robert said. His emphasis was on "we."

Him, me and God.

You better get your act together, Jehoshaphat, you're coming too.

✳   ✳   ✳

A cloudburst hit as soon as we reached our car. I put my head in my hands and sobbed. Robert was near tears also. He reached over and put his arms around me.

"I'm glad Mom went back before we saw Dr. Santala." I took the handkerchief Robert offered and blew my nose. "At least she didn't have to go through this part!"

"You're still going to have to tell them," said Robert.

"I will. I will be OK," I assured him and myself. "It's just hard right now. Let's go home."

It was one of the quietest trips that Robert and I have ever made. The 130-mile trip was a vacuum. Conversation was brief.

"I have to be at work Friday," he said.

"I know. I was thinking Phyllis could take me."

"That's a good idea."

"I didn't know they gave chemo and radiation at the same time," I said.

"I didn't either."

"I guess I better get a wig."

"He said your hair might not fall out."

"*Might*—I think I better get a wig."

"Do you think I'll still be able to work?" I said.

"Well, we'll just take it a day at a time."

"I suppose I should tell them all this so they can plan a work schedule."

"Tell them first thing in the morning."

"I will."

I wanted my blankey and my bed. Robert looked like he could use a blankey too. When we got home, I went to my hovel bed. He crawled into bed with me under the covers. He hung onto me tightly.

"We'll be OK," I said. "God is going to be with us. Remember my Jehoshaphat chapter? He said, 'The battle is not yours, but God's.'"

"I know," said Robert. "Let's pray." We prayed. Then he left me to rest.

I slept a little while. Then I woke up, scared out of my skin.

Back at the Cancer Center I had given Fear a key to my mind. She was staking her claim as I lay in the dark. I could feel my hair falling out. My stomach was churning like a merry-go-round. Terrifying visions were projected across my brain. I saw them digging my grave. My family and friends were crying. I exchanged places with the women in the wheelchairs. I was the one sitting with a turban around my bare head.

I was lying in a recliner in the window room at the Cancer Center.

I wanted to jump up and run straight to Robert.

"You can't do that," a voice whispered. *"He needs his sleep. Besides, you'll scare him to death!"*

OK, Lois, get a grip here! This is a Satan attack! Pray! "Lord, stop this insanity, please stop these pictures!"

They didn't stop. Over and over again. Visions of funerals, graves, sickness, dying. Instant replays of suffering and pain.

"Naturally your prayer won't work," contin-

ued the insidious whisper, *"Your faith is just a joke!"*

I was crying now. *Maybe I could go to Carol. No, Robert would hear the garage door open. He'd wake up and be really worried.*

I willed myself to lie down. I counted sheep but they kept turning into ugly woolly monsters.

"We've got you now! Listen to us . . . all of us. Your God is abandoning you. We have ammunition you can't fight. You're losing ground fast! This is where the plot thickens!"

After about two hours of this, I jumped up and practically ran to our bedroom. Robert was sound asleep on his side of our king-size water bed. I went to him and shook his arm. Standing there in my long blue nightgown, I nearly scared him to death—waking him from a sound sleep.

"What's the matter?" he mumbled as he rubbed his eyes, "Are you all right?"

"No!" I boo-hooed. "I'm so scared!"

He lifted me up into our bed. "Now what's wrong?"

I told him about all the fears, crying harder as I talked. "I thought I could just pray and they'd go away. Why won't my prayers work? I didn't want to wake you. I don't want to scare you."

"Listen to me. Listen to me, Lois."

Now he was crying too. "I was beginning to think you didn't even need me in all of this," he said. "I was thinking you could handle it all on your own. I was feeling shut out."

He went on talking, holding me tightly to him. "We need each other through this. You and me and God. Don't ever be afraid to wake me up or tell me you need me. I want to share this with you."

It was a long time before either of us went back to sleep. One thing for sure, I wasn't going back to my hovel bed until daylight!

Finally Robert whispered, "Lois, are you still awake?"

"Yes."

"Let's pray again."

Fear was evicted from my mind that night, taking all of her dreadful dreams with her. I don't remember the words Robert prayed. But I never had such a terrifying attack of those dreadful nightmares again.

For both of us, that night was the end of our solo flights. We pledged our vows anew: For better or worse; for richer or poorer; in sickness and in health, we are one.

The two of us—alone together . . . with God and His servant Jehoshaphat!

"Ye shall not need to fight in this battle: set yourselves, stand ye still, and see the salvation of the LORD with you, O Judah and Jerusalem [Robert and Lois]: fear not, nor be dismayed; to morrow go out against them: for the L ORD will be with you" (2 Chronicles 20:17, KJV).

Prayer Needs

We appreciate your prayer support more than you'll ever know and it is our prayer that God blesses you as you have blessed us during this time. We are over-whelmed with His love and care and mercy. We are praising Him. Psalm 27:4-6

We are claiming the victory of the bat-tle as reported in Second Chronicles chapters 19 and 20. Please read that to see how God used many people together as *He gave the victory!!*

Radiation treatments are at 10:30 am each day Monday through Friday for thirty treatments which should finish about April 1. Pray for our travel, drivers, weather and no complications. These treatments are at the Northern Rockies Cancer Treatment Center in Billings.

Chemotherapy is more complicated and will be more difficult physcially and emotionally. (The battle on the moun-tain.) Lois will take two drugs by injection twice a month and one drug by mouth for fourteen days.

And this continues for six months so should end by August. The problem that can arise is blood count to get too low and infections, etc, can change schedule so pray that we can rebuild and renew as needed. As you pray, I pledge to eat right, get rest and drink lots of fluids which is critical to the treatment.

Thanks for sharing this with us. We'll try to keep you posted on changes. Again may God bless you! He certainly has pleased us!!

Robert and Lois

Chapter 11

The Pilgrimage

"I think God just gave me an idea," I said to Robert as we were driving home to Colstrip a week later. "What if I had a different person drive me to Billings every day for radiation?"

"I want to drive you as much as I can," he said.

"Oh, I know. But you can't do it every day. I just think it would make the trip less boring if I had a different person driving me, besides it would be a test to see if I really have thirty-five friends!"

"Would you ride in their cars?"

"No, they could drive our car. I would just be the passenger. I can rest while they drive."

"Well, it might be a good idea. Would you only want people from church?"

"No," I was getting excited now with the whole idea. "I could just put the word out and see who volunteers. And there would be rules too."

"Rules?"

"Yup, rules. First, no one could have two turns, except for you, of course." I reached over and patted his shoulder.

"What're the other rules?"

"Well, I don't want anyone that drives really slow—that would drive me nuts! And those are the only two rules I can think of right now."

"We don't even know if you're going to be driving every day. What if you get sick?" Robert asked. "What if you decided to stay in Billings? What if the roads get bad?"

"Well, then we could change the rules!"

The idea was great. I settled back in my seat thinking about the trips ahead of me. *Dr. Lamm said I would have thirty to thirty-five radiation treatments. Robert will probably drive me at least five times. That means I need about thirty drivers. Hmmmm.* Soon I was sound asleep.

I woke up as the car turned into our driveway. "So what do you think?" I said.

"About what?"

"About the drivers? Is it OK with you?"

"Whatever you think," he said. He was saying that lots lately.

"OK, I am going to do it!" I was in my Lois-on-a-mission mode. Whenever that happens, I shift into accelerated, single-minded action. Like a bulldozer. "I am going to set up a schedule."

And I did. It was such a blessing. As the trips were counted down and the miles added up, I knew for certain that the idea had not been mine. Only God could have formulated such a brilliant plan! It didn't take long for the schedule to have names penciled in. I only planned a week at a time. Just in case complications arose.

Robert was reassured when he saw his name on the days I would have to stay in for chemo treatments. He approved of my stormy-weather backup drivers too. These were well-seasoned drivers with four-wheel-drive vehicles that had volunteered to be ready whenever there were icy roads.

Pete, one of my best friends, was my driver on my third trip. He's a Christian brother who was a friend to our boys, particularly Ross. He has been a special mentor for my Christian walk. And we love to talk! Which I guess we were doing too well. It took a few seconds for the siren noise to interrupt our conversation.

Sure enough, the flashing red and blue lights and the siren were for us. Pete came back to the car after "visiting" with the patrolman in his car for several minutes. He had a pink slip in his hand.

"Did he give you a ticket?" I asked.

"Yup."

"Didn't you tell him you were taking a cancer patient for radiation?"

"No, he just said I was going seventy-five in a thirty-five mph zone. I didn't say much after that!"

I was indignant. "That road construction sign has been up every day and no one's even working there!"

"That doesn't matter. I should have slowed down."

"How much was the ticket"

"I don't know. I have to go see the judge."

"Yikes," I said. "In Colstrip?"

"No, in Billings."

"Great . . . then you can have two turns!"

He smiled. "OK, that's a deal."

So Pete got two turns. He never told me what that ticket cost. He wouldn't let me pay it either. I think it was pretty expensive, but I sure did enjoy his two turns anyway!

"Where did you go to high school?" I asked.

"What?" Robert was my driver of the day. We were two miles out of Colstrip on our way to Billings for my radiation and chemo treatments.

"Where did you go to high school?" I repeated. "See, right here I always ask my drivers where they went to high school. It gets the conversation going." He gripped the steering wheel a little tighter.

He thinks the radiation is affecting my brain. I smiled to myself.

What a grand time these trips were! Every trip was different. I never tired of the daily 260 miles. I got better acquainted with people from work and from my church.

"I went to high school in Miles City at Custer County High School," answered Suzanne Brown to "the question." She was my driver of the day.

We attended the same church, but I confessed I really didn't know much about her. "What was your early life like?" I asked.

"Kinda laid back, weren't much an old country gal like me didn't lack! Kinda early to rise, kinda early in the sack! I thanked God I was a country gal."

I laughed.

"Seriously," she said. "My life was good. I grew up on a farm with four brothers, two sisters and parents committed to one another. I was very secure in my family and had a fairly normal life. Yet although we attended church regularly, I felt a desire to be nearer to God."

"When did you actually come to know Jesus Christ?" I changed positions in my seat, putting my feet under me.

"I committed my life to God on September 8, 1973, when I was in eighth grade. At least that's what my diary said." She chuckled. "I remember responding to an altar call yet nothing really changed in my life. But I believe God saved me that night even though I didn't know it. Through a series of events over several years, the Lord brought me to a personal relationship with Him and gave me assurance of my salvation. Do you want to stop at the rest stop?"

"No, if you don't. Just keep scooting on. How has God changed your life? And do you want part of my orange?"

"No, I am OK. God changed my life in several ways, including improving my self-confidence, purifying my lifestyle and changing my attitude about the Bible. I used to think the Bible was the most boring book around. Then one day while I was attending a Christian camp, I picked up a piece of paper lying in the lounge. At that time I collected sayings. The paper I picked up had neat sayings on it, and I read everyone of them, clear to the bottom of the page where it said '1 Corinthians 13.' Wow! What a shock! The Bible *was* interesting. It told how God had changed me on the inside. I didn't even know it, yet He chose a unique way to show me how He'd changed me. God is faithful. Is this the exit we take?"

"Yes, and thank you for blessing me today with your life."

And it continued. My drivers enriched my life. Nan Taylor drove on a Thursday. I wasn't feeling well. It was a low day on my "feelings chart." But she talked and I listened.

"I was searching for something more in my life," Nan said. "I married at eighteen, thinking this was what I was searching for. I had my first child at nineteen, knowing this had to be it; I got pregnant again at twenty-one, still looking for the answer. My aunt shared Christ with me after our son Trent was a few months old. I immediately accepted Him. That faith was tested very soon. Trent went into a coma at eighteen months and was diagnosed with insulin-dependent diabetes. We came close to losing him."

"I didn't know diabetes was discovered that young. He seems to be doing good now?"

"Most of the time. How are you doing?"

"OK, I'll just lie back and keep listening. How did God change your life?"

"I'm no longer searching for the answer of life, but searching for how to serve Him. I realize that people, husband or children, cannot fulfill my life. The Person of Jesus Christ is the only One who can do that."

Ginger Reimers walked down to my house on her driving day. Besides attending the same church, she and her husband were our neighbors. When she got in the car she said, "OK, so are you going to ask me where I went to high school? I heard about your question!"

"OK, smarty! So satisfy my curiosity. I know you came from Minnesota. Were your family Christians?"

"My mother was a Christian, so I remember going off to church once in awhile on Sundays and at Easter. I remember Easter because of our home movies with us in our Easter bonnets parading up and down the sidewalk before an old 8 mm camera!"

"I bet you were cute!"

"I also remember an impatient father with a fiery temper who would get home from work and take off again to the bar if we were being too noisy!"

"That probably isn't a precious memory. . . . How did you get to meet Jesus?"

"Well, one night when I was in second grade, some cousins invited my family to special meetings at their church. We went, and the hand of God touched my father. That night Dad accepted the Lord Jesus as His personal Savior. I watched God change some things in Dad's life overnight, others He's still transforming."

"I have goose bumps right now! Then what happened?"

"In watching the miracle God performed in Dad's life and knowing that if Dad needed a Savior . . . so must I, I realized I had to make peace with God too. One night upstairs in an old two-story white stucco house this eight-year-old girl walked from her bedroom down the hall into her parents' room and knelt by their bed. I realized that I would never be good enough on my own to deserve heaven—"

"Some people are lots older before they come to that understanding," I interrupted.

"I knew I was indeed a sinner, needing a Savior. I prayed with my parents that night to accept Jesus Christ as my personal Savior and to cleanse me from sin. He did just that and has been faithful to me ever since that day!" She glanced over at me. "Am I boring you?"

"Never! Keep going. I don't even have to ask you the questions!" I laughed.

"Church and its fellowship became a big part of our lives. I remember getting a Bible for Christmas from my grandma when I was in third grade. I loved looking up the Bible stories and reading them for myself. I also loved the memory work. Do you want me to keep rattling on?"

"Yes, I'm really being blessed! We turn at the Twenty-seventh Street exit. The gas station is on the right."

"It's just that there are so many things God has done for me and taken me through in my life, it's hard to pick out just one or two. Thanks for listening."

"Well, just hold your place. We have the trip back, and I want to hear more." And we did just that.

"As the next few years rolled by, I experienced the death of many kids my age. Life and death were very real to me, and therefore so was the importance of my eternal relationship with my God."

I nodded, thinking how God works differently in each life.

"So throughout the years being teased about not being able to do this or that because of my 'religion' never bothered me a bit. Actually I believe it strengthened me and helped me stand for the Lord. The concept of unconditional love and acceptance was overwhelming—the fact that belonging to Him as His child was all I truly needed. He alone is big enough to provide for all our needs—physical, spiritual and emotional. My self-worth lies in who I am in Christ, not in human eyes, but my God's!"

"You should share your testimony at Christian Womens Club! I know many women lack self-worth these days. I cannot imagine what it would be like to have cancer and not know God!"

"Only when we look to God alone to meet our needs for love, acceptance, self-worth and belonging, can we truly have healthy relationships with people around us. What joy and freedom I found in knowing what God's Word says about me is true no matter what people may say."

"I think I needed to hear that today. I appreciate you!"

"The Bible says, in John 8:32, 'the truth will set you free.' . . ."

"And the truth has blessed and encouraged me! What a trip!"

So day by day I got radiated—and uplifted. Every driver had a different approach to life—and to driving. Most loved to drive our slick gray Thunderbird. I had the supplies I needed stuffed in every corner in case of emergency, but there never was one. Only a few close calls and one encounter with the patrolman!

Not going with any "slow drivers" really got around. One driver was slow, and I was chomping at the bit the whole trip. When I got to the Cancer Center and went in for my treatment, I told the nurses and technicians, who were all good friends by now (and curious and interested in my drivers), that instead of praying for my driver today, I was praying for me!

"What happened?" said Robert, my rad tech, as he adjusted me on the table. "Did you get another ticket?"

"Fat chance of that when you're going fifty-three!" I complained. My mood was lousy. "I should have an attitude treatment instead of a radiation treatment," I said as I got up off the table. "See you tomorrow!"

Putting my bra and shirt back on in the change room, I prayed, *God, please forgive me! How fast we drive is not important. Change my attitude, please!* I walked out into the waiting room to tell my driver I was done.

There stood Kevin and Kelli, our kids from Seattle, with a huge bouquet—a dozen red roses! And a teddy bear! I bawled! What a surprise! And what a terrific day for a surprise. *Thank you God* . . . I rode back with my designated driver. They followed behind us. On the trip back it didn't matter how fast we drove. My soul was flying in the clouds!

During my last week of treatments I did more flying. I flew in for my treatment. Bill

Mayo wanted to be one of my drivers. His wife, Leona, said, "Lois, you don't want him to drive you! He'll go fifty-five the whole way."

A week later, she called me. "I have an idea how Bill can take you, and you won't have to ride with him!"

"And how are we going to do that?" I asked.

"He'll fly you!" Bill has a private flying school and has taught flying lessons and ground school for several years. I had flown with him before.

"That would be terrific!" I said. "Let's do it!"

So for my thirty-second treatment, I traveled in class! Leona went along for the flight. Since I didn't want to disturb the "driver" I said, "OK, Leona, how did you meet Jesus?"

"Listening to a story in children's church I realized I needed to ask Jesus into my heart. The leader prayed with me after children's church. That was a long time ago!"

"Now watch your talk," I retorted. "You're younger than me. I'll soon turn fifty."

"God has been with me through lots of things. Like bringing me to Colstrip, taking me away from my comfortable Christian college gang. . . . I had to learn how to deal with non-Christians, to love them and be concerned about their eternity. Mother died when I was young, then my father spent four-and-a-half years in a coma, and I was ill during my teens. Through all that I have seen God work! That verse in Ecclesiastes chapter 3, I think, says 'a time to be born, (3:2, KJV) and a time to die.' I may not understand God's timing but I know it's under His control and He knows best!"

"Amen to that! I'm learning the same thing!"

My coworkers, neighbors and friends from the community and people from our church all volunteered to drive. I had more volunteers than I had days. I looked forward to each day and wondered what experiences I would hear about. My boss at work, Mike Holzwarth, was one of the stormy-weather drivers. So our trip was on icy roads on the day he drove. He canceled the burgers-and-shake part of my schedule. We had a fun lunch at a Mexican restaurant that day.

I have fond memories of every trip and driver. God blessed me in some way through each one. I remember being with my friend John Bleth, from work. His mom had died from cancer just a few years earlier. I think it was painful for him to be reminded of her ordeal. But he drove, and I learned how a family member feels about cancer. It was good for me to hear.

Many times family members question the treatment choices. Is this the right one? Should they be doing something different? Most of the time these questions are not voiced to the patient. The family member goes through some lonely times of agony.

Later I asked Paul Hoefeldt how he felt as Pat battled cancer. He told me about trips home after leaving Pat at the hospital. "I pounded on the steering wheel. I yelled at God. I was angry and then felt guilty for being angry. I went over every detail. What could we do differently? Why Pat? Why not me? Why now? Why? Why?"

After talking with John and Paul, I decided to keep the door open with my family members so they would feel free to discuss their feelings honestly with me. I prayed that God would comfort them in their dark hours as He had comforted me.

As the last week of radiation treatments approached, I got another great idea!

"Robert," I said to him that night while we were eating supper in my hovel. "I have another great idea!"

"Now what?" he said. "You decided to do your radiation over so you can have more trips?"

"No, no thanks! But it has to do with that. How about throwing a party for all my drivers? We could use the church basement . . . that would be fun!"

"Are you sure you're up to that?"

"Sure. I could get people to bring stuff. Everyone is always asking what they can do. Lisa could bake one of her beautiful cakes . . . let's do it!"

It was Lois-on-a-mission mode again. One idea followed another. I invited my folks to make the trip down so they could meet all my drivers. Ross and Marla came from Glendive. I went to the local sheriff's office and asked to speak to our area highway patrolman, Jeff.

"Wouldn't it be fun if you pulled up in your patrol car, sirens going, and arrested all these people for using up too much of the highway?"

He looked skeptical. "I'd have to check with my commanding officer."

"Well, do. I'll call you back later. This is going to be great!"

He called back in two days. "I got the OK. Now just exactly what am I supposed to do?"

"I think you should give everyone a ticket. I'll make them up—"

"I can get you a copy of the real thing if you want it."

On one of our chemo-rad trips to Billings, I broke my promise not to shop. I picked up race-car invitations and red and blue award ribbons. I got two big "grand prize" ones too. I wrote out all the tickets giving awards for the trip with the most bathroom stops (Pastor Mike); the slowest trip (Patti Kimmet); the scariest (Nan, when we slid to a stop at the train crossing and narrowly missed getting hit by the cross arm); the tallest (Bill and Leona for the plane ride); and ones for all the rest of the drivers with various captions.

All but three of the drivers came to the party. We had a great dinner. My friends and family pitched in. Jeff, the patrolman, came on cue, and together we stood at the front of the group handing out the tickets. What laughter! Pete got one of the grand-prize ribbons for the most exciting trip. "And I have no idea what that trip cost!" I quipped.

There were tears when I gave the other grand-prize ribbon to Robert. Everyone knew how hard my cancer had been for him and how much he was supporting me emotionally and physically. I cried too and hugged him. I thanked everyone for all they had done for me. Words couldn't convey my gratefulness.

"Could you show me the upstairs of your church?" Mabel asked me. "I've never been in this building."

"Sure," I said. "Follow me." People were standing around visiting. I wouldn't be missed.

We were just finishing up our tour when Sharon Burton came up. "Come back downstairs, you two."

I got to the second from the last step when I heard, "Surprise! Surprise!"

The church basement had undergone a transformation. From my "Driver's Roast" it was turned into a surprise fiftieth birthday party for me! I bawled. Then for the next hour, I opened silly gifts and rotten gifts and precious gifts. The party was complete with a birthday cake (Lisa had been busy!) and black balloons and crepe paper.

When I went to bed that night, I cried some more, overwhelmed with how blessed my life continued to be, how grateful I was to my family and friends and how God continued to pour out His blessings on me through others. But that is getting ahead of my story.

We need to go back to February for the first radiation and chemotherapy appointments.

"Just who is writing the words for this play? The script doesn't say cancer makes friends and there's fun along the way!"

Drivers

February

```
20, 21 ...Phyllis Rowe
24 .........Ginger Reimers
25 .........Pete Mellbom
26 .........John Bleth
27 .........Sharon Buckner
28 .........Robert
```

March

```
2 .........Toni Dobear
3 .........no treatment
4 .........Sharon Burton
5 .........Son, Todd - snow
6 .........Suzanne Brown
9 .........Russ Eide
10 .........Pete Mellbom "to see the judge"
11 .........Robert
12 .........Sharon Buckner
13 .........Cheryl Richards
16, 17 ...Carol Lands "stayed over"
```

March

18.........no treatment
19.........Mike Holzwarth - snow
20.........Robert
23.........Darlene Sharp
24.........Patti Householder
25.........Patti Kimmett
26.........Marilyn Watson
27.........Mary Pattison
30.........Susie Wollan
31.........Daryld Watson

April

1.........LaRae Kaski
2.........Nan Taylor
3.........Fly - Bill & Leona Mayo
6.........Hugh Broadus
7.........Pastor Mike
8.........Robert

Chapter 12

You Drive, I'll Hold the Bucket

"Yes, I have a bucket. I have soda crackers. I have towels. I have 7-Up. I have my blankey. I think I'm all prepared."

"Do you want me to drive over to your house?" my friend Phyllis asked. She had been chosen by Robert to take me to Billings for my first official radiation treatment (number one of thirty-five) at 5 p.m. We would spend the night at the Billings Inn, then she would go with me for my first round of the six months of chemotherapy.

"No, I'll come pick you up," I said. "I have all my stuff in our car. I can still drive, you know!"

We had a good visit on the way in. We laughed about the card she had just sent me. I had gotten a card from her and Jim at the hospital. The day before I had received another card. Written on the bottom was: "I heard you say you had received six cards from Carol. I'm now realizing that this is a more-than-one-card illness. So here is my second. Love, Phyllis!"

We checked in at the inn. It's a popular place for people receiving medical treatment. It's across the street from the Deaconess Hospital and the Billings Clinic. My appointment for chemotherapy was at 3 p.m. the next day at the Clinic. My radiation appointment was in thirty minutes at the Cancer Center just up the street. We decided to walk.

Phyllis was delighted with the Cancer Center duck pond. "Looks like God is paving the way for you," she said. My arm was more than a little sore from the Olympics of the day before—the simulation day. But I had confidence that God would see me through this first treatment, and the rest of them.

Phyllis said, "Let's pray before you go in." We had a time of prayer. Praise God for friends who don't just pray before meals and at bedtime!

"Lois, you can come with me," nurse Pauline said. I was ready. I wanted to get started on the offensive. Zapping cancer cells was the battle plan for me and Jehoshaphat.

Following Pauline to the dressing room, I said to myself, *Number two in 1942 . . . room number two. I remembered!* I donned my battle uniform, a pea-green, wrap-around style, short cotton robe. I just had to take my shirt and bra off. They only needed the top! Then I went to sit in a chair in the Rad Club waiting room.

The treatment went well. Very well. The technicians introduced themselves as Joe and

Robert. They put my personal styrofoam mold on the steel table in the large room. Then they had me slip off the pea-green robe and lie back in the mold. They were very careful about getting me positioned just right. My left hand was to be on my forehead. The thumb of my right hand was tucked into my waistband. They set up the linear accelerator. I named it the Zapper. I could see styrofoam molds of different shapes on shelves on two sides of the rad room.

The room had a calming tan wallcovering. Someone had hung an airplane made of pop cans in one corner. The accelerator was a futuristic looking machine. Everything sparkled like it was new. Dr. Lamm was there making sure the program he had set up for me was being carried out according to his plan.

"Now lie very still," technician Robert said. "We have a video camera and sound system to this room. If you feel nervous, you can talk to us and we can talk to you." When they walked out of the room, it sounded like a five-ton door was being shut. I thought of when I toured Alcatraz.

All right, Lois, this is it. I was ready. I started to sing. I wondered if Jehoshaphat was listening.

Here we are, Lord, in Your presence, lifting up holy hands in one accord—whoops—I can't lift my hands up.

Before I could choose another song, the doors slid open and Robert was back with Dr. Lamm and Joe.

"Now the next angle," he said. Dr. Lamm had decided to radiate not only my left breast, but the areas surrounding my axillary nodes and those at the left side of my neck.

"If the cancer traveled to your axillary nodes, I'm not going to rule out involvement in your upper lymph nodes," he said. I was glad.

My surgeon, Dr. Brown, had told Robert and me that in the 1960s, a group of physics graduate students at Stanford University built the first linear accelerator to be used for clinical purposes. "The patient was a two-year-old boy with retinoblastoma, a cancer of the eye," he said. "He had already lost the other eye to cancer. As a result of this machine, the eye and the boy's sight was saved.

"One of those graduate students, who went on to earn his Ph.D. and devote his career to high energy physics, was Karl Brown, my father. The clinical achievement remains a fond moment in his life as a physicist. It is easy to get lost in the minutia of basic research. To see one's efforts in action for the good of man can be a rare event for one in basic research.

"While my father has spent essentially all of his career at Stanford University, he did take a leave of absence to work on further refinements of clinical linear accelerators. His area of expertise is beam optics. To get an electron beam from one end of a linear accelerator to the other requires focusing and bending of the particles with specialized magnets. The design of the magnets and their organization in series is the job of a beam optics expert.

"You may have noticed on the linear accelerator that a wide arm hangs out over you with the beam coming out of a port on the undersurface facing you. In order for that to occur, the beam has to make a 270° turn. That sequence of magnets was designed by my father and patented by Varian Associates for whom he consulted. Without that bend, the machine would have to be, well, linear. You would have been postioned at the end of a machine that looked like a telescope. Imagine how tall the ceiling would have to be!

"Thought you'd like to know that more than one member of my family cared for you," Dr. Brown had told me.

Zap me wherever you want to, I thought. *We're in a battle here, you know.*

"Out so soon?" said Phyllis. "I haven't even started reading my book. I was so busy watching the ducks . . . and the people. How was it?"

"Not bad," I answered as we went out the door. "I can see why John Williams laughed when I said I thought I would take my music tapes in with me. There isn't time!" We went out to supper. Then we went to Hennessys to look up the wig department. I had the card from my Hennessys' angel in my purse.

"They look like dead squirrels!" Phyllis said.

"Look at this one!" I said.

"That's not bad . . . look at this! How about blond? It would be a total makeover!"

"No thanks! I sure don't see any with just a little gray in the front. Do you?"

One by one, we eliminated every one. None passed the test of being held up to my head. None had gray streaks in the bangs.

"You know what I think?" I said. "I think I'll just get my old wig out of my costume box. It looked great on me in the '60s. What's wrong with just having Les fix it up? Maybe she can even put some gray in it?"

"Sounds like a good idea. Won't hurt to try it," agreed Phyllis. "What have you got to lose?"

We giggled. "Just your hair, I guess . . . !"

Rad number two was crossed off my list the next morning at 10:30. The staff was so friendly. They all called me by name.

We made our way to the second floor of the Billings Clinic way ahead of time. I led the way to the oncology department waiting room. Phyllis was carrying my tape deck. In my purse was a bottle of 7-Up and a towel. Just in case I got sick right away. The waiting room seemed different. The puzzle was still there—a little more complete, but not done yet. The people sitting in the chairs were no longer future negative images of myself. They were other fighters. Other survivors.

"Now what do you want me to do?" asked Phyllis. "Do you want me to go in with you or stay here and pray?"

"You can come with me and pray!" I said.

"Lois? Did you get your lab work done this morning?" nurse Kathy asked as we followed her.

"Yes, I did."

"Remember to have them use your right arm, not your left."

"Yes, I will," I promised. I had read all the literature about the risk of lymphedema. In big letters it said, "Do Not Permit Blood Specimens to Be Drawn from This Arm."

"I'm not an easy person to get blood from," I told Kathy. "My mom isn't either. We have little slippery veins, I guess. Every time my mom gives blood she ends up with black and blue blotches all down her arm . . ."

Shut up, Lois, I said to myself. *You don't have to give her your whole family history!* To Kathy I said, "As usual, when nervous, I blab!"

"She does!" agreed Phyllis, who was now carrying my tape deck, my coat and my purse. All I had was my faithful notebook. Into one of the window rooms we went. I figured I would take the recliner, since I was the "star."

"You're really getting the hang of this!
Now we can get this production moving.
Places, everyone!"

Kathy left the room. "Let's pray together," said Phyllis. We had barely said amen when

Kathy returned with a syringe and two little tube-like vials of liquid on a tray. "Do you want your earphones on now?" asked my faithful friend.

"No, not yet. Wait until they get the IV running," I said.

"What IV?" asked Kathy.

"Don't you put this stuff in with an IV?"

"No."

"I thought everybody got chemo with an IV," I said thoroughly confused.

"Some drugs are given intravenously. Others by injection and others orally."

"Oh."

"Dr. Santala has put you on CMF. You'll be getting the methotrexate and fluorouracil, we call it 5-FU, by injection into your veins. The cytoxan is a tablet." Kathy took my right hand looking for a vein. "You do have little veins . . . here's one."

I noticed her gloves. "Is it hard getting used to doing all this while wearing rubber gloves? I have a friend who's a physician's assistant. She says it takes some getting used to. It's for your own safety though, that's—"

"You'll feel a little prick."

I forgot she didn't answer my question. *Well, Lois, here it goes, welcome to the world of throwing up!* I thought. *I better start singing.* But instead I tried to feel what I was feeling.

"Does it sting?" asked Kathy. "Some patients feel a stinging sensation."

"No, it just feels cold. I can feel it going in my veins."

"That one is done," she said. "Now the other." She pulled the little tube off the needle, leaving the needle in my vein.

She attached the other little tube and slowly released the liquid into the needle.

"How do you feel?" asked Phyllis.

"I feel fine." We were done in less than thirty minutes.

"Dr. Santala has given you a prescription for some nausea medication. The directions will be on the bottle. Take it if you need it. It isn't good for you to feel terrible. Some people try to get along without it. We give it to you so you won't suffer with the nausea."

As we walked out, I saw Dr. Santala standing at the nurses' desk. I still didn't like him. He was smiling and laughing. The nurses were talking with him like he was a regular person.

OK, give him the benefit of the doubt. Maybe he was just having a bad day on Wednesday. Maybe one of his patients died . . . now there's a happy thought, Lois! I scolded myself. We walked to the elevator. I had a cotton ball taped onto my hand.

"How do you feel now?" Phyllis was doing her part well. Robert would have been pleased.

"I still feel good."

"Do you think we should get the prescription filled before we leave?"

"Yes, let's. I think that would be a good idea."

I waited in our car while Phyllis went to the drug store. The bucket was on the floor by my feet. I put a towel across my lap. The 7-Up was in the cupholder between us.

"Now you just lie back and rest," she said as we pulled onto the interstate highway.

"I still feel OK."

I repeated that phrase every twenty miles of the trip home. "I still feel OK." I was really surprised! I did feel OK. We listened to a Gordon Jensen tape my friend Bruce had given me.

"I can feel it going through my bones," I told Phyllis. We had been on the road about an hour. "It feels weird."

"Do you feel sick to your stomach?"

"No, I don't. I feel fine. Tell me about what God has been doing in your life lately. I'll just lie here and listen."

"Sometimes I'm overwhelmed. He has literally changed who I am. Remember my foul mouth and the bitterness and anger I was carrying when we first met at the ceramic shop?"

"Uh huh, yes, I do!"

"Now I know peace and a quiet trust in the Lord regardless of life situations! He has changed the lives of my children and has turned them around. He has set me free from many things, like my mouth!" We both laughed. I still felt fine.

"Let me tell you about cleaning at Pluggie's house a few weeks ago. I saw a dozen or so vine-ripened tomatoes on the counter. I pondered what to do with them and where to put them. At the same time, I eyed them for a popper. You know, one you could just pop into your mouth. Alas, they were not mine to eat. To remove the temptation I quickly looked for a basket to put them in. Just at that moment my little lady called from the living room, 'Phyllis, do you like tomatoes?' In my heart I was hearing the voice of the Lord much plainer than Pluggie.

" 'Yes,' I answered the little lady.

" 'Well, I have more than I know what to do with,' she said. 'Why don't you take them all home with you?'

"Why didn't I just ask her for a tomato when I knew she would have said yes?"

"I don't know, but I bet you're going to turn it into one of your Phyllisophosies!" I said.

"I am. God used this to show me He sees our temptations and He will provide a way out. And second, He will give to us if only we ask. And third, I could see also that many times we try to reach out in our flesh to grasp at a small portion of the blessings in life that God wants to freely pour out in abundance!"

"Wow! Good lesson!"

"How do you feel?"

"I still feel fine."

Phyllis pulled in our driveway. "We can get you to bed and then Robert can take me home," Robert was beside the car before she shut off the ignition.

"How do you feel?"

"I feel good."

"Did you throw up?"

"No, I feel fine . . . It must hit later."

Robert and I prayed together before I went to bed for the night. Every night we prayed for my doctors, our family and the concerns of some of our friends.

"How do you really feel?" he asked with his hand on my shoulder.

"I feel fine, really."

Just before I went to sleep that night, I reached up and gave a lock of hair a tug. It didn't come out.

When I woke the next morning, I felt a little queasy. Robert came into my hovel the minute he heard me stirring. I don't think he slept that night. "How do you feel?"

"Queasy. I feel a little queasy but pretty good otherwise."

"I'll get one of those pills." I took the pill. I knew I didn't dare question Dr. Olmstead.

"It worked out good having your chemo on Friday. That way you'll have all weekend to rest," he said. I knew that was not just a statement; it was an order.

Phone calls came throughout the day. The first phone call was from my folks. "How do you feel?"

"Really good," I said. "I was a little nauseated this morning, but I took one of the pills they gave me, and I have felt fine since."

"You keep doing just what they tell you," said Mom.

"And you rest!" said Dad. "You don't have to be up running around."

"I won't. I feel fine." And I still did.

"We're praying for you and so are all the people at church here. They're all asking about you."

"Tell them I love them, and I love you too! I really am doing fine."

I stayed in bed all day. Resting. There were lots of phone calls and some visitors throughout the day. Pastor Mike came over. We had a good visit and a time of prayer together.

We had decided—my personal medical committee: spouse-doctor Robert, real-medical-person Carol and me—that I would take my cytoxan pills in the evening right after I ate supper. The initial reactions of my body to the drug could take place while I was asleep. I took the three pills at 7 p.m. Then I went to sleep and slept well.

Sunday morning my stomach was upset. Not throwing-up upset. Just sickish. I took the nausea pill before I ate breakfast. Soon I was feeling fine again.

"Are you sure you want to go to Sunday school and church?" asked Robert.

"I'll go to Sunday school, and if I get feeling icky you could bring me home. How does that sound?"

"OK" But he was pretty skeptical.

Everyone at church was glad to see the person they had been praying for.

"How do you feel?"

"I feel good."

"How do you feel?"

"I feel good." Over and over and over and over again. "I do really feel good." I was most amazed of them all.

"How do you feel?" asked Cheryl, our pastor's wife.

"I feel good. I felt a little icky this morning when I first got up but I took a pill for that. Now I feel good . . . and I still have my hair!" I joked only half in jest. I found myself checking my head often.

"Well, you just aren't going to lose your hair!" she said emphatically. "I am going to pray that you don't!"

Chemotherapy—Application

1. When you go for your first appointment be sure someone goes with you—a family member or friend. When you actually walk through the doors of a *cancer center*, it can be a traumatic time.

2. Look around you for blessings. If you trust God, He will prepare the way for you. Maybe for you it will be a painting on the wall or a view from the window or your favorite color on a chair. Maybe it will be a flower arrangement—with your favorite

flower in it. But you must have your eyes open.

3. Let your prayer-support team know the exact day and hour of your appointment and remind them to pray for you.

4. Read all the brochures on chemotherapy that are given to you and if they aren't given to you at the time of surgery, ask for them from the American Cancer Society or your doctor.

5. Remember this is part of the introduction in the new chapter in your life, and God is there with you. You can write this story with humor, intrigue, anticipation, sorrow, pity, adventure, tragedy, suspense, poetry or song. It's really up to you.

Bible References

Isaiah 42:16
Psalm 100
Psalm 63:1-8
Psalm 68:19
2 Chronicles 20:22
Matthew 11:28

Psalm 25:5
1 Peter 2:9
Psalm 59:16-17
Luke 11:13
Matthew 6:33

Chapter 13

Does This Journey Take Many Pages?

Several years ago we took what every family would consider a dream vacation. We went to California. We planned for months. Our itinerary included Marineland, Universal Studios and Hollywood. We made plans to swim in the ocean. We would see the zoo. We would visit museums and Olivera Street. Of course we would visit Disneyland. We sent for tickets. We poured over all the brochures of things to see. Our trip would be two weeks long. Every day we would visit new exciting places.

The morning of departure finally arrived. Our fifteen-foot Roadrunner camping trailer was packed to the hilt. The three boys, ages fifteen, twelve and nine, piled excitedly into our new yellow Wagoneer. Robert tooted the horn twice, a family tradition meaning "Wagons Ho!" and down the road we went.

We made it to West Yellowstone, about five hours from our starting point, before we heard

"When will we get to Disneyland?" for the first time.

That six-word refrain soon took top priority over our normally most-often-heard statement on family trips: "I got to go to the bathroom. Now!"

We viewed the majestic Tetons.

"When will we get to Disneyland?"

We went over historic Donner Pass.

"When will we get to Disneyland?"

We saw a desert for the first time.

"When will we get to Disneyland?"

We toured a walnut farm. Saw orange groves along the highway. The traffic. The cities. The Californians! Nothing swayed the all-consuming mind-set of the crew in the back seat.

I gave a lecture on enjoying each day. No change. We threatened to throw the next person asking *the* question overboard. Nothing worked—except driving into the parking lot at Disneyland. Thankfully it was everything they had dreamed it would be. We had a marvelous time at Disneyland. None of us will ever forget it.

But those boys sure missed a lot of grand adventures on the way to their destination. I have never forgotten that lesson. Because I do it myself many times. One goal in mind. One mission to accomplish. One job to complete for the day. One possession to save for. One accomplishment that will gratify my needs. One way for God to answer my prayer. Every other thing becomes secondary—just an irritating detour.

Now there is time for single-mindedness. We need goals and destinations. But we dare not let one objective become an obsession. We might miss all the "sights" along the way. Like an intimate, honest, soul-searching conversation with a friend. Unusual birds enjoying a worm dinner on our lawn. A leaf bud unfolding before our eyes. The giggles of our four-year-old grandson as he shares a jar of 79-cent bubble stuff. The delight in hearing by phone how well this year's cattle drive went for my folks.

Serendipities, the faculty of finding valuable or agreeable things not sought for, sprinkle my days. Moments of joy. Blessings from God. Fleeting passages of life, enriching jewels to be treasured. I determined in my heart, by the grace of God, to live each day of my life to the fullest. I tried to listen to God's direction for each situation. I read His Word faithfully to get strength (spiritual food) for my soul.

Because I determined in my heart to keep my eyes and ears open, taking time to listen, to see, I didn't yearn for Disneyland. I enjoyed the sights along the way. I prayed for God to enable me to do so. That decision has made my life to this point full of adventure.

"Do we have a surprise for you! This play will not have just a one-week run. It's going

to have a successful run, like My Fair Lady.
It will be interesting to see how you, our
lady, fare after a few weeks!"

With Carol's help, I made some decisions on a plan of action for my life and cancer. As a physician's assistant, she had many experiences with cancer patients, as well as in her own family.

"You must be *extremely careful* about germs," she told us. "Your white blood count will more than likely hit bottom. Your resistance to disease will be nil. Any cold or flu bug can be life threatening to you while you are undergoing treatment. Rest is vitally important. You need to save your strength to build healthy cells. Some are destroyed through the chemotherapy and radiation."

> Anticancer drugs can affect normal tissues also, because they act on any rapidly dividing cells in the body. The normal cells most likely to be affected are those in the bone marrow, gastrointestinal tract, reproductive system, and hair follicles. Most normal cells are able to recover quickly when the treatment is over.
>
> *Chemotherapy and You*, U.S. Department of Human Services (Publication no. 91-1136)

She was right. I read the brochures that were given to me. The necessity of staying healthy and getting lots of rest was strongly emphasized. My healthy cells were called into the battle also, whether they wanted to participate or not. So I made a list in my notebook (naturally!):

1. I would rest.

> a. as soon as I got home from work—to bed
>
> b   all evening going would be curtailed
>
> c. my new lifestyle would be rest, rest, rest
>
> d. I would not argue when Robert said, "Rest." (That was dictated by him.)

2. I would eat wisely.

> a. lots of fresh vegetables and fruit
>
> b. cut out fats and some sugar (The "some" was dictated by me.)
>
> c. heavy emphasis on calcium and vitamin C

3. I would live as if a "leper." (This was dictated by Carol but the leper part was my idea.)

> a. wash hands hundreds of times a day
>
> b. do not touch mouth with hands ever
>
> c. refrain from shaking hands with people
>
> d. touch NO door handles, door knobs

or any other publicly used items (Sometimes it was real circus on this one.)

e. if around sick people, wear mask

f. white blood count low—go into isolation

4. I would view trips to Billings as medical trips not shopping trips. (Guess who wrote that one!)

5. I would accept help from others.

6. I would sing. Me and Jehoshaphat.

"OK, guys, I got it," I said. "I'll do my utmost to follow these rules, cross my heart, hope to die (whoops), if I tell a lie."

Robert and Carol looked skeptical. But our plan of attack was established. And I was "established" according to Second Chronicles 20.

Careful daily records were kept. I recorded my feelings along with the medical information each day. I graded my general well-being feelings on a scale of one to ten: ten was feeling great, one was feeling like spaghetti boiled too long. Most days I was at the five or six level. I had a few low days, but the number of high days was more than the low days.

One of the main stresses of cancer was how my up-and-down feelings just threw me bonkers. One day I was a ten, and the next I was a one. Or I went from a ten to a six. Or a five to a nine. Or a seven to a three. Or . . . the more treatments I had the more my feelings fluctuated. I would have felt much better if someone had told me ups and downs were normal.

Our routine followed the same pattern every day. Only the weekends provided variety in my schedule.

6:30 a.m.—Get up, bathe and dress

7:00 a.m.—Call my folks

7:15 a.m.—Eat breakfast, usually cooked cereal, fruit

7:45 a.m.—Robert leaves for work, I drive our car to my driver-of-the-day's house or they come to our house and leave their car

8:00 a.m.—Leave for the two-hour trip to Billings

9:00 a.m.—Be around the Hysham Hills area. Eat orange or apple

9:50 a.m.—Stop for gas at station three blocks from NRCC

10:00 a.m—Arrive at Northern Rockies Cancer Center

10:15 a.m. —Have my radiation treatment

10:45 a.m.—Stop at drive-in for turkey sandwich and milk shake

11:00 a.m.—Travel home (two hours)

1:00 p.m.—Arrive at my job at Colstrip Community Services

4:30 p.m.—Off work, home to nap in hovel

    5:30 p.m.—Supper together in hovel
    6:00 p.m.—Write in my journal, read my
             Bible
    7:00 p.m.—Take cytoxin pills according
             to schedule. Carol comes over,
             visit, pray, games, videos
    8:00 p.m.—Prayer time with Robert
    8:30 p.m.—To bed, listen to hymns on
             tape

On the Fridays I had chemo this schedule varied. Most often Robert took a day of vacation from work and drove on those days. We stayed in Billings the entire day. On several chemo-days my folks met us in Billings. (They live two hours west of Billings.) They went with me also for my injections. On chemo-days I reported for lab work at the Billings Clinic at 8 a.m. So we often traveled the night before and stayed at the Billings Inn.

Excerpts from my journal follow to give you an example of my thoughts and feelings.

2/16—was wonderful to praise the Lord. Pastor spoke on sure foundation of Jesus. Amen and Amen.

2/17—back to work, got lots done, brain still works! Evening we were on panel for teens Sweetheart Party. It was Newlywed Game. We lost!

2/18—worked at training Annette some more. She will take my place when I am gone for treatments. Everyday I get comfort from caring people, cards and letters, etc. I would like to *feel* more spiritual, closer to God. I feel steady and sure that He is in all this—I just don't *feel* saintly or angel-like, but I do feel very content, at peace.

2/25—started period, took nausea pill and felt good. Pete got a ticket seventy-three mph in thirty-five zone! wonderful trip, got tattooed. Thank God, we got through that. At least I don't have to worry anymore when I shower. M. Watson, supper, two pills.

2/27—felt good but slept little after 2:30 a.m. Saw Dr. Lamm, good visit. Karrie cleaned house, had hair done, wig is ready. Karrie brought supper.

3/11—Again I will sing praises to the Lord, for He has blessed me with His everlasting love. He has taken the fears and the concern and hid them under His wings. I know His eyes are ever on me. His angels are preparing the way ahead of me as He directs. I praise Him for the faithfulness and labors of love of the saints.

3/16—You know what I really enjoyed about Sat., Sun. and today? There were activities, going out to breakfast, going for a milk shake with Cheryl, a garage sale, church, visiting the Baptist church. And then today in Billings, visiting nurse Pauline's house to see her Victorian bathroom and shopping for mine. I felt like me again, the pre-cancer person, but of course I'm the cancer-person now, so I can *appreciate* being out, being with a friend like Carol, who was so *giving* and unselfish, and finding just the right stuff!! How can I say thank You, Lord? You bring sunshine into every day.

3/18—No treatment, Zapper broke (radiation machine), SNOW, 'spose God knew it would snow today . . . wallpapered bathroom, had coffee break with guys on CCSC crew. Rested in afternoon, Todd came to visit. Thank You, Lord.

4/4—I didn't sleep at all, underarm is real bad, burns hurt. This is worse than the worst sunburn I've ever had. I think I'll ask the elders to pray for my burned arm.

4/25—Bones feel weak, weird. WBC was 1.8 yesterday, but felt great the day before—weird. Brown and Santala say "lower cy dose."

5/8—the effect cancer has on a marriage is devastating. I feel we have one of the closest marriages around and if it is rough on us, woe to others.

Day by day, hour by hour, we walked through the doors before us with some good days and some bad days. My pen released my feelings on page after page in my journal.

Just how many pages was this journey going to take? For certain, Robert and I and God and Jehoshaphat were on a pilgrimage. Only God knew the number of pages needed. And I had to trust Him.

Date	Work	Comments	Feel
Jan			
31	Fri 0	FINA, yearly physical, breastlump found	10
Feb			
1	Sat 0	Ladies Rally Blys, calling fam, friends	10
2	Sun 0	Church, Anointed by Elders, James 5:14	10
3	Mon 0	8 am EKG, XRay, 9am BROWN, Noon surgery "malignant"	1
4	Tues 0	Painkillers (ha!) my armpit hurts	2
5	Wed 0	Feel better, Amazing! Out of hospital	4
6	Thu 0	125 cc drain, 5 perc, period started	4
7	Fri 0	99 cc drain, 4 perc, lots vist, slept good	5
8	Sat 0	60 cc drain, 2 perc, arm better, shower	5
9	Sun 0	55 cc drain, 1 perc, went church, ate out	7
10	Mon 0	10 cc drain, 1 perc, breast leak, arm hurt, tired	5
11	Tue 0	25 cc drain, 1 perc, spoke at Valentine banquet	6
12	Wed 0	BROWN, tube out, tape off, OUCH "TININO"	5
13	Thu 8	Back to work, pap test OK, Thanks Lord	6
14	Fri 8	Arm Exer, OUCH, tired - played house	5
15	Sat 0	Stayed in bed, rest	5
16	Sun 0	Church, led worship service, rested	9
17	Mon 8	Work, arm exer, hurt/spoke at youth cl	8

18	Tue 8	Thinking Lots about Cancer deaths	8
19	Wed 0	LAMM, SANTALA-DAY OF RECKONING-HARD	5
20	Thur 8	Emotional, worked, then to Blys for red	7
	Work	Comments	Feel
March			
7	Sat 0	Breakfast out, taxes, movie, tired rest	6
8	Sun 0	Church, few mouth sores, but doing good	8
9	Mon 4	Felt tired in evening	6
10	Tues 2	Pete> judge! long wait rad mach broke	8
April			
9	Thu 4	Sores re real bad, stayed home am.	5
10	Fri 8	1st 8 hr day, felt good 'cept armpit	8
11	Sat 0	Ran lots of errands, had to nap in pm	8
12	Sun 0	Gave party for drivers, "roasted them" Then surprise!! They roasted my bday.	10
13	Mon 8	Arm and breast are sore today	7
14	Tue 8	I am 50 today! A golden oldie-tired	6
15	Wed 8	Underarm sore, booster sunburn peeling	6
16	Thu 8	Wild case of energy! Feel good	8

Chpater 14

The Skirmishes

In a real battle, there are skirmishes where the two opposing sides do hand-to-hand combat. The final outcome of the battle may depend on the result of the skirmishes. In each war the skirmishes vary.

So it is in the cancer battle. Each cancer patient reacts differently, physically, spiritually and emotionally. The same drugs react differently in different bodies. One victorious life-long Christian will face tremendous depression; another will develop more interest in her surroundings. One cancer victim will fight the enemy head-on; another will want to curl up and die. One may want everyone to know their struggles; another will keep them private.

Just as the cure for cancer is so elusive, so are the paths that each patient takes. What is most difficult for one is a breeze for someone else! I did not struggle with being physically sick as some of my friends have. I did not lose all of my hair, which is a horrifying experience for both men and women. Yet there were parts of my cancer battle that were really difficult for me. This chapter deals with those. My skirmishes!

How Do I Know?

There are lots of things in this world I do not understand, like gravity, how we can see television pictures sent from the moon and how my computer stores all these words for me as I type them.

One thing I have always understood though was me. My body. After fifty years you get pretty confident about the way your body reacts. I know if I stub my toe on the corner of the bed, it's going to hurt. And hurt a lot. If I have a virus, I will get a fever, headache and maybe throw up. If I take antibiotics, my body responds. Sooner or later, I feel good again.

If I wallpaper a room in my house, climb up and down a ladder and bend over the tub soaking the wallpaper, I will barely be able to crawl out of bed the next morning. My muscles are reacting to my one day of physical labor.

I know me. I have grown accustomed to my body. As a matter of fact, maybe it is the only thing in the world I really know and can count on. Except for the Lord, of course. He made me this body.

"Hey you! You have an error there. You should say the only thing you used to count on. You won't be trusting your body anymore. After all, look how your body deceived you. We've been at work in your body a long time, maybe even five years. You didn't know it, did you? All the time you were walking around thinking everything was fine, we were busy at work. You were really duped. You did breast self-exams every month. You went for annual physicals. Your blood pressure was perfect. You felt great . . . and all that time we were engaged in building your tumor! Fooled you, didn't we? Not so sure of the ol' body right now!"

No, I am not. I do feel differently about the body that houses me. Sometimes it feels foreign. Alien. Cancer proved to me that I do not know what is going on inside my body. The evidence came in the form of X-rays and surgery and pathology reports. Sometimes I feel betrayed by the very thing closest to me.

I know that the real Lois is the me inside this shell. When I die, the me that I am will go to heaven. The Bible references at the end of this section explain how I know this. But while I am here on this earth, this body is my home. I can't trust my body like I used to. Especially since my surgery.

As I undergo chemotherapy, my white blood count (WBC) drops as the toxins work at destroying new forming cells. When the WBC is extremely low, I am vulnerable to germs, bacteria and viruses. But I cannot tell by how I'm feeling what my white blood cells are doing. I have to wait for my blood test. Sometimes when I feel the most energetic, my WBC is very low. When I feel very tired and listless, I am usually making blood cells . . . at least then my WBC goes up! It is disconcerting not to know what is going on inside of me.

"We really got you wondering, don't we? Are we still conducting building surveys somewhere in your 'house'? Have the chemotherapy and radiation gotten rid of all of us, or are we hiding somewhere in your liver, behind your knee, in that sore spot on your neck? You can't tell for sure anymore, can you?"

Discovering that cancer cells have been busy in your body can make you feel alien to your soul's own habitat. It's a weird feeling. At times I feel the separation of "me" and my body.

This is not all bad, because according to God, "we" are not our body. But we tend to forget that since our body enables us to breathe and live and function here on earth. Our personality, our self-esteem and our self-confidence are often products of how we look. The shape and condition of our body is important to who we are. Advertisements tell us all the things we can have and be if we use this perfume or deodorant or toothpaste. . . .

You control your body. You can dress it up or trim it down. You can beef it out with exercise or shrink it in with diet. And if you don't like it the way it is, you can surgically get it pinched in, tucked up or flapped under! You are in control.

"We certainly took that control away, didn't we? Bet you won't ever feel that confident again. This is one of our most effective ways of pulling you down and getting you to run scared. Good stunt, huh?!"

And that became a constant skirmish. Dealing with those scary words, "took that control away." Over and over again I had to go back to Second Chronicles:

Do not be afraid or discouraged because of this vast army. For the battle is not yours, but God's. (20:15b, NIV)

You will not have to fight this battle. Take up your positions; stand firm and see the deliverance the LORD will give you. . . . Do not be afraid; do not be discouraged. Go out to face them tomorrow, and the LORD will be with you. (20:17, NIV)

How Do I Know? Betrayal—Application

1. Don't let this betrayal feeling freak you out. Your body did not betray you. Cancer is not sneaking around uncontrolled in your body if you are actively fighting it. You and your physicians are on the offensive.

2. Recognize the vast healing power of our Lord. He created the human body with a remarkable defense system. The very fact your cancer was discovered is evidence that an invasion has not gone undetected. The human body God gave us is unlike anything man has contrived!

3. I found healing and comfort in the touch of another human. When someone put their hand on my shoulder, I felt relief. When a friend held my hand, I felt they were touching "me" in this body. A pat on the knee or a touch on my arm eased my feeling of separation.

4. Sometimes, lying in bed, my husband laid his head over my shoulder right above the lymph node surgery area. Or he carefully (very carefully) laid his hand on my breast over the lumpectomy incision. I felt the strength from his body and his touch pouring into my body. It was so tender and so comforting.

5. Remember right now your body is a battle-field. There has been an enemy attack. But you are fighting back. God is enabling you to be strong. People have regained control of their countries by combat against ene-mies. The opportunity to rebuild and heal comes after the battle.

6. As in every other aspect of cancer we have discussed, don't keep these feelings to your-self. Talk to your doctor, an oncology nurse, a family member or friend. Write down how you are feeling. Write how the fears af-fect your emotions. Ask someone to pray with you about them.

Bible References

HEAVEN
2 Corinthians 5:1
Revelation 22:14
John 14:12

BODY
1 Thessalonians 5:23
1 Corinthians 6:19-20
Luke 12:22

FEAR
Psalm 34:4
Psalm 118:8
Isaiah 50:10

A Hot Flash Is Not a Late-Breaking News Bulletin

Many chemotherapy drugs put the body of a woman into menopause, referred to as "chemically induced menopause." After a few weeks of chemotherapy, my list of enemies from cancer changed from cancer cells, radiation and chemotherapy, to cancer cells, menopause and menopause.

Night sweats and mood swings were my two biggest difficulties. A flannel nightgown, socks on my feet and a comfy quilt had been my lifetime night habit. Numerous "little talks" over our thirty years of marriage covered "his" open windows while I froze in bed, enduring hurricane blasts of frigid air.

A husband of a cancer patient must have flexibility and patience:

> "Open that window wider!"
> "Get those covers off of me!"
> "Could we have a little air-conditioning, please?"

But if you have been there you know the next phase three minutes later:

> "Shut that window!'
> "I need more covers!"

Buying light cotton pajamas was my first remedy. I took two blankets off the bed. (And kept the quilt at the end of the bed for the freeze-phase.) I tried to learn how to cope when the equator heat wave was detonated by some sneaky hormone-fuse lighter in the middle of the night. I tossed covers off, threw my leg out over the edge of the bed and in a few minutes the "blast" was over.

The hot flashes were impossible to anticipate. Different times, different places, different emotions. I could never figure out what triggered them. Once when I was sitting in a chilly lecture hall, I tried to get one to come on. I couldn't and nearly froze for an hour. At work, I could be totally involved in a spreadsheet, and "wham!" I was hit with a body temperature over a 100 degrees. Coworkers got used to me running out the door to breathe in some cold Montana air . . . only to rush back in and put my sweater on, freezing from the inside out!

The hot flashes not only affected me but Robert as well. For months the hot flashes continued. The perspiration ran off my forehead. My bangs got wet. In the middle of the night, my pajamas were so soaked with perspiration I had to change.

"I can't stand to put my hand on your body," Robert said, awakening out of a sound sleep. "You're so hot."

The mood swings affected him more than the hot flashes. I felt bad about the ups and downs of my moods as I dealt with hormonal changes. My moods made no sense.

In desperation, I asked my friend Sharon Buckner to attend a menopause seminar with me held at the Deaconess Women's Health

Center in Billings. I thought I might get some help there. All of the workshops were on the usage of estrogen, something I could never take since my cancer was estrogen-positive. (I had thought that was "good news" back then!)

In one workshop, a sample copy of a Canadian newsletter, *A Friend Indeed*, was passed around (*A Friend Indeed*, Box 515, Place du Parc Station, Montreal, Canada H2W2PIk, 514-843-5730). In it I saw a previous newsletter in November 1990 had been on "Chemically Induced Menopause." When I got home I sent for that newsletter and several others. It was the most helpful information I found on the subject.

Since that time, much progress has been made in dealing with chemically induced menopause and the availability of hormonal therapy for women who cannot take estrogen. My husband says, "Praise the Lord!"

Only he knows how awful my emotions tumbled during those months—well, he and me and the Lord. Along with his love and support for me during the treatment months, I am thankful that he forgave me for some awful times. I hated myself most of all and didn't know how to stop or control my moods. Maybe someday doctors will have a pill for that!

Hot Flash—Application

1. Ask your oncologist on the onset of symptoms what is available for you. I was in error

during my treatment. I figured the cancer was his concern, the hot flashes and mood swings were mine.

2. Go to your local women's health clinic. Check out new publications on the subject. Your local library will have updated material and news releases on the latest treatments available to you.

3. Recognize each woman has different menopausal ailments. Your first thought will be, *It is more cancer!* when, in fact, it may just be another timing adjustment in your hormones.

4. Through it all, ask the Lord to touch this area of your body as well. Ask Him to control your mouth. I had to do this constantly. And be quick to ask forgiveness of those you offend. Guilt is not a desirable companion.

5. Make an investment in clothing. Just as you would if you were going through pregnancy, a change is necessary in attire. Get things that are in layers—jackets and sweaters can easily be taken off or put on.

6. Keep your sense of humor! There are lots of good, humor-filled books on the market about menopause. Instead of crying, laugh! Those around you will be thankful.

Bible References
Psalms 120 and 121

Now Where Did I Put It?

Another side effect had me a little more concerned. I have done a lot of dumb things in my life. As a matter of fact, the opening line for many of my speaking engagements is, "What I am here to tell you is that in spite of all the dumb things I do, God loves me anyway!"

So to think that I might not be able to *think* was disconcerting. I had to pay more attention to details. I also decided that after all the dumb things I had done, probably nobody would notice a change!

Even before chemotherapy was in my life, I sometimes lacked concentration. One day I went to the laundry room and prepared to do my washing. I started the water in the machine and then went into the bedroom to get our dirty clothes out of the hamper. Two hours later I walked by the washer. Sure enough it had gone through the whole cycle with no clothes in it. Somewhere between the washer and the bedroom I got sidetracked. I told my husband I had run the washer on a "cleaning cycle."

Another time a friend came by my house to pick me up to go out for coffee. She went out the door first and headed down the sidewalk. I thought she was taking the long way around to get over a large snowdrift in front of our house.

I had my knee-high snow boots on so I just plowed through the drift. I got in the car and sat down.

Hmmmm. I never noticed their upholstery is the same as in our car, I thought as I waited for my friend. *They even have a tape case like ours.* Then my brain engaged. I was sitting in our car on the passenger side, seatbelt fastened. My friend was sitting in her car behind ours, wondering what in the world I was doing. (In my defense, both cars were blue!)

And that isn't all. We joined another friend for coffee. After visiting awhile, she said, "Lois, why are you wearing only one earring?" Grabbing my ear, I discovered she was right. I had no earring on one ear . . . but the other ear had an earring with two backs on it! I made a mental note right then to watch myself more carefully.

I'm always getting up to go get something in the house and when I get there, I can't remember what I came for.

I've found my dishwasher detergent in the refrigerator, my car keys in the silverware drawer and the milk carton sitting in the cupboard beside the plates. I have been afraid I didn't pay my phone bill when I try to make a phone call and don't get a dial tone—only to discover I left the phone off the hook in the basement after my last call. I got in a tizzy about my mental state and how ditzy I was going to be after all the chemotherapy drugs went

208 BREAST CANCER AND ME

through my system. But then I conferred with a few friends and felt better.

Maybe it isn't the chemo.

Another acquaintance finished her day at work. Glancing out the window, she waited for her husband to pick her up. He was usually right on time. After waiting thirty minutes her patience wore out. She called home. "Where are you?" she asked. (We tend to ask dumb questions when we're upset.)

"Right here," her husband said. "Why?"

"You were supposed to pick me up! I'm waiting!"

"Honey," he said sweetly, "I can't pick you up. You have the car."

Another friend told me in confidence that her husband called from the bedroom, "Hon, where're my socks?"

"In your drawer where they always are," she answered.

"No, they're not," he said. "There's a package of hamburger in there, though."

She didn't miss a beat. "Well, then look in the refrigerator. Your socks must be in there." They were.

Maybe it isn't the chemotherapy. Maybe it isn't the menopause. Maybe it is just normal!

Hang Me on a Coat Hook, I'll Sing from There

Sleeping has never been a problem for me. I

have always been a morning person and followed that old adage, "Early to bed, early to
rise." But cancer treatment changed all of that.

At first I thought it was worry or fear that
was keeping me awake long hours in the night.
However, after committing every single thing I
could think of to the Lord, I was still awake. I
asked people to pray for me. I was still awake.
Finally checking with Dr. Santala, I found out
that sleeplessness is a common side effect of
cancer treatment. Patients undergoing radiation or many of the chemotherapy protocols
find they cannot sleep.

It is one of the most discomforting side effects. You want to go to sleep. You want to rest.
You are bone-tired. But your brain will not shut
down. In talking with other cancer survivors,
the most common comment was, "I thought it
was just me."

Now some individuals in treatment are being
given sleeping drugs that are safely compatible
with their chemotherapy drugs. Just another
wonderful advancement in the cancer fight.
Maybe I wouldn't have felt like a loser in that
skirmish if I was going through treatment today.

Concentration Loss and Sleeplessness— Application

1. We cannot blame all of our mental foibles
   on chemotherapy and our cancer involvement. But certain chemotherapy drugs do

have an effect on one's concentration. That was evident to me. I love to read. Yet I couldn't manage to read for more than a few minutes at a time. I learned to be honest when friends offered to loan books to me. Be honest with those around you about your particular changes.

2. When awake in the middle of the night, I watched travel videos. *National Geographic* has created several of these which were loaned to me by a friend. Your local library would have copies.

3. My favorite help in the long hours of the night came from Moody Bible Institute. They put out wonderful videos on God's creation. One I found particularly good was titled "Perfect Peace." It was given to me by my folks' church family. I also enjoyed the Moody Praise and Worship Series. These were uplifting for my soul and perfect for my concentration limits. (Contact Moody Videos, Moody Institute of Science, Chicago, IL.)

4. My Bible was a source of encouragement. Reading my chapter from Second Chronicles reinforced my goals. Praying also brought comfort and courage in the dark nights.

5. My friends Marty and Cheryl were going through treatment at the same time I was

getting treatment. We made a commitment to be available for each other—in the middle of the night. Cheryl and I both had phones by our bed; Marty often spent his nights in his recliner in the living room. When one of us had a need to talk to someone "with skin on" in the middle of the night, we could call each other. Find a friend who will make that commitment to you.

Bible References

I found only one verse to relate to this phase of treatment.

"Where there is knowledge, it will pass away!" (1 Corinthians 13:8, NIV)

All Alone on an Island?

After you have gone through all of the treatments for breast cancer, you would expect relief and happiness. There is cause for celebration. But this does not happen with most cancer patients. And I was no exception.

The day of my last treatment I cried on the way home. I cried because I would miss the friends I had made at the Cancer Center. I realized I would miss the special attention they gave me. That thought made me cry because I was so self-centered. Then I cried because I was crying. Surely I should be glad to be out of that place! Why wasn't I happy? When Robert asked me what was wrong I couldn't answer. I didn't know what was wrong.

The feeling persisted for weeks. I felt like I was on an island. Alone. How could I tell anyone my feelings? They would think I was crazy.

Everywhere I went people hugged me and congratulated me on being done. "I'll bet you're glad that's over," they'd say.

"Sure," I would say. But I'd think, *Why don't I feel glad?*

I felt orphaned and those feelings overwhelmed me. It was a rough time in our marriage. I wanted to return to normal life. Life before cancer. But I didn't know how.

My strength was low. I decided to start walking around the lake every morning like I did before cancer. The first morning I couldn't make it up the hill on the path around the lake. So I cried my way home. Other days I told Robert I was going to clean the house after work. But when I came home from work I had only enough strength to crawl into bed and cry some more. *What's wrong with me?*

Then the little voices returned.

"They didn't eliminate all of us. We're still in here. Hiding. Hiding. Hiding."

Robert and I had a terrible fight. He was putting clothes from the washer into the dryer. I came into the room and pushed him aside. "This is my job now!" I yelled. "I'm not an invalid. I'm not sick. This is my responsibility. I don't want you to touch these clothes!"

He backed up in stunned hurt. "I'm just trying to help." He reached to hug me.

I pushed him away. "I don't want your help. I want to be well! I want to do things again. I want to be back to normal. I want . . ." I started wailing. "I just want to have things be like they were before!"

He led me to the couch in the living room and sat beside me. I couldn't get control. I knew I was a creep but I couldn't stop.

"No one understands," I cried. "I don't even understand my feelings. I should be happy! I should be thankful! Why can't it just be like it used to be?"

"Because you're still weak," he said. "You don't realize how much your body has lost through all of this. It's going to take a long time for you to get your strength back. You're going to have to be patient. I'm doing these things for you because I love you. I want to help you, Lois. Do you understand?"

He handed me a handkerchief.

I blew my nose. "Nobody tells you how to deal with life after cancer! I don't even know who I am anymore. I'm not the same person. How can I ever be the same person again after all this?"

"Neither of us will be the same as we were before. We can't. And that's not all bad. We have gone through a lot. God has given us many blessings. Focus on that. In many ways we're better than we were before."

"I don't feel better right now," I sniffed. "I just feel like I'm out on an island all by myself. And I'm fat." I had gained fifteen pounds in the past few months.

"You are not fat! You'll lose weight when you get to walking again. And even if you don't lose it, it doesn't matter. I love you. You are not out on an island by yourself. I won't let you. I'm with you. God is with you. It's just going to take some time. You're more worn out than you realize. Now let's go in the bedroom and get you ready for bed. You need your rest."

I followed him obediently. He was right. I was so tired. And he was also right that I wasn't alone. The next evening I scanned the brochures and cancer books I had collected. Some alluded to emotional problems following treatment. Other people had experienced weight gain (or loss) during those months. *Maybe this is just like the postpartum thing after having a baby, the "baby blues." I just have to be patient.*

Since patience doesn't come easily to me, the next few weeks were punctuated with moodiness, despair and crankiness. I searched the Scriptures, finding solace in the Psalms. I again experienced sleepless nights. I replayed the videos that comforted me during treatment. I made a list of people I wanted to communicate with and wrote cards. Somehow writing thank-you notes to doctors, nurses and friends helped me close the door on my treatment phase. In a few weeks I was on my island less often.

The island faded in the distance when I realized that I would never return to life BC, before cancer. Making that discovery gave me peace. I was not the same person. I never would be. This was a new beginning. A new me. It was my choice if I was going to accept the new me. I learned to like the new me, a breast cancer survivor filled with hope and looking forward to the future. I left the old me on the island and walked on.

Aloneness—Application

1. Feelings of aloneness are common among the women I talk with who have gone through cancer treatment. Being aware this can happen will lessen your feelings of guilt and anxiety. You are not alone.

2. Find a breast cancer support group if you have not done so already. Continue to go as long as you want to. Switching roles from the treated one to the survivor will help you and others in the group. Don't stop going because you feel as if others think you should. Some of my friends found comfort by attending months after their last treatment.

3. If you cannot overcome feelings of aban-
   donment, call your nurse and share your
   feelings. If necessary, see your doctor and
   talk with him about your feelings. Ask for
   his recommendation for follow up.

4. Undoubtedly your body will go through
   physical changes. You will gain weight
   (all those milk shakes) or lose weight.
   The appearance of your breast will
   change. Whether you have a mastectomy
   or a lumpectomy, there will be transfor-
   mations to deal with. And the tatoos. Try
   a new hairdo or enroll in a health club.
   Your doctor can give you names of busi-
   nesses that will counsel you about breast
   forms and choices. Try whatever will
   help you feel better about your appearance. Just don't try everything at once. Be
   patient!

5. Deal honestly with your fears. Make a list
   of your feelings. Examine each one. Determine which ones are realistic. Confer with
   your doctor or nurse. Go to your library or
   bookstore. Read books that deal with life
   after cancer.

6. Pray. God has not stopped listening to you
   just because you're done with your treatments. I found writing out my prayers
   helpful at this time. Read God's Word. The
   Psalms were a real comfort to me.

7. Maybe this is the time to write about your cancer experience. Put your thoughts down in a journal. Leave it as a treatise for your family or write it just to God. Or write it as a help to someone else. Maybe it will even turn into a book like this!

Lois Is So Strong

Another skirmish is not peculiar to cancer patients, but my cancer experience highlighted the temptation. Sometimes when we feel on top of things or when others express their wonder and amazement at our strength in tough circumstances, we can be tempted to believe we are great.

Our adult Sunday school class was learning about the importance of lifting each other up. Now encouragement is wonderful, and we should do more of it. On this day though, it was a skirmish.

Bill Mayo, the teacher, said, "Tell us some way that someone has encouraged you the last few weeks."

One after another, class members shared experiences.

Next it was Carol's turn. I was thinking of what I would say. *How can I put into a few short words all of the blessings that have been showered on me?*

"Lois has been an encouragement to me," Carol said. "I know what it's like to go through surgery. I don't think I handled it very well.

But being with her and watching her trust in the Lord has been a very good lesson for me. She is so strong."

A lump in my throat made it difficult for me to swallow. Robert lovingly put his arm around me and squeezed my shoulder.

"Right! Sure! You are strong. All we need to do is get you thinking you can whip us. We can let you have one little victory. Then we'll hit you with some heavy ammunition. We'll see who has the lead in this play! Go ahead. Take your eyes off that God-stuff and you're a goner!"

"I guess you all know what I am going to say," Robert said as he patted my shoulder. "God has been so good to us. I want to thank all of you who have helped Lois." Then he got that grin on his face that warns me I'm in for it. "And just keep those dinners coming! I never knew how good home-cooked food was!"

In the midst of the laughter, I jabbed him in the ribs. *Ouch, my arm still hurts.*

"I can't begin to say what all the encouragement has meant to me during the last few weeks. . . ." I lifted my hands toward the class. "You have all blessed us more than you will ever know."

"Little do you know . . . it is downhill from here! Just wait until the news of us gets old, then we'll see who is left blessing you!"

Another chorus of "Amen!" and "Praise the Lord!"

It was Cheryl's turn. She is the wife of Pastor Mike. "I just want to say I went over to see Lois this week, to encourage her. . . ." She burst into tears. Sniffs, coughs and nose-blowing soon followed from others. I grabbed for Robert's hand. "I just wanted to say how much she encouraged me," Cheryl continued. "She is so strong, and she just really encourages me."

I slid down my pew and gave Cheryl a hug. "Your visit helped *me*. I was so glad you came."

But as I slid back to my warm spot beside Robert a big old dark cloud descended. I felt cold. I felt like a teeny-weeny ant in a room full of giants.

Lord, I can't do this. I can't. I can't. I can't. I am not strong! *I can't do this. I am not strong! I don't know how to do this cancer stuff!* I debated standing up and screaming to the whole class, "I am not strong!"

But I didn't do that. These people were expressing their thoughts, not mine. God was using me to encourage others. I had prayed for that, hadn't I? It was going to be me and ol' Jehoshaphat. I grabbed for my notebook and, as I typically do, I wrote in my journal what I could not say out loud. And peace came as thoughts spilled into words across the lines. . . .

This is part of what I wrote:

Lois is not strong—God is strong.
Lois is not strong—people are praying.
Lois is not strong—other women have gone through this.
Lois is not strong—BUT GOD IS!

Skirmish—Application

1. Recognize there will be skirmishes along the journey.

2. The success of an ambush is in direct proportion to the surprise of the attack.

   a. Each of us have different vulnerabilities

   b. Falling into despair is as easy as falling off a cliff when one is camped on Cancer Mountain

3. Remember word attacks can cause only superficial wounds, not life-threatening ones. Put on your bulletproof vest. Make sure it is the Word-proof quality. Be aware that words spoken are not necessarily the same as words heard.

4. People mean well. Put yourself in their place. They are concerned. They care

about you. They want to offer solace. The lack of sleep, the hormonal changes, the physical toll of your particular treatment all cause strange reactions in your system. Your emotional reactions may not be up to par.

5. When skirmishes come in the form of sneak attacks, such as self-pity, discouragement, depression, anger and irritability, *run, don't walk* back to the original battle plan: Second Chronicles chapter 20.

Chapter 15

The Blessings Came Down . . .

*And when they began to sing and to praise, the
LORD set ambushments against the children of
Ammon, Moab, and mount Seir, . . . and they
were smitten.*
　　　　　　　2 Chronicles 20:22, KJV

Jehoshaphat, I wonder if you were as as-
tounded and humbled as you stood on that
mountain as I am as I sit at this keyboard? I wonder if the awe of God's power on your behalf, a
mere speck on the seashore, overwhelmed you
as it does me? Did any words of gratefulness you
uttered seem insufficient? Did you feel alone?
Unable to express how thankful you were?

Did you have a wife who walked with you
through those days, encouraging you, supporting you, doing tasks you should have been doing, pouring out love that covered all your
failings? Did you have a mom and a dad who
shed tears before God on your behalf and
wished they could be in your place so that you
would not have to suffer?

Did you watch the singers that marched out in front of the enemy lines and marvel at their faith as I did about those who walked the cancer walk with me, like Marty and Cheryl? Did you have army captains that believed in you like Dr. Santala, Dr. Lamm and Dr. Brown believed in me? And chaplains to teach you and advise you like Pastor Mike and Pastor Walt advised me? Were there encouraging runners beside your chariot like my nurses who encouraged me?

Who drove your chariot? And who cooked your meals? Who washed your clothes and cleaned your house and took over all your community and work responsibilities while you waited upon the Lord for victory?

Did you cry sometimes because there were no words to express to God what you felt? Did you feel God reach down and touch you when you were feeling discouraged and afraid?

Jehoshaphat, do you know that your testimony and the choice you made to follow God and believe in Him and be obedient to Him made a difference in my life in the twentieth century? And Jehoshaphat, could I look you up when I get to heaven? I want to hear you sing!

* * *

"When I say there were blessings in my cancer experience," I asked Robert, "what comes to your mind first?"

"Gigi's meals! And God answering my prayers! And lots of other things. Do I have to make a list?"

"Nope, I was just wondering how I could ever list them all for my book."

"Oh, you mean you're 'Counting your many blessings,' naming them one by one?"

"Yes, and it's impossible."

"Well, just start writing and it will come to you. I'll pray."

I hugged him. "You always do. That's one of my favorite blessings! I'll start with Gigi since it was your favorite!"

✳ ✳ ✳

Right after I got out of the hospital, Gigi Batie called and said, "I want to bring supper to you on Tuesday night." She's a fantastic cook, a mother of two teenage boys and a busy lady with lots of activities in the church.

"I would love it and I *know* Robert will. I'll tell him you're bringing supper next Tuesday and he can write it on the calendar."

"No, I don't mean just this next Tuesday. I'll bring supper to your house every Tuesday night."

"You're kidding!"

"No, I want to do it. See you Tuesday."

And she did. Gigi cooked supper for us every Tuesday night. Delicious meals. On

pretty plates, sometimes with a note, a flower
or some other special treat. Many times she
brought enough for two meals. Robert
thought he was in heaven! When I finished
my radiation trips, I wrote her a note and
thanked her for the blessing she had been to
us through her meals.

"We're not done yet," she told me. "You still
have four more months of chemotherapy!"
And for the next four months, *every* Tuesday
night we got a treat from Gigi Batie's kitchen,
often with her husband Dan or one of the boys
being the deliveryman. What a blessing!

Blessings in the form of cards and letters
poured down. I keep the cards in baskets beside my computer desk. Jan, the daughter of
my high school friend and college roommate,
Sharon Buckner, mailed many cards. First, she
sent an elephant card that I still have on the
wall in my hovel. It says, "I am pulling for
you." Week after week, Jan sent cards. Later I
found out more about her motivation.
Throughout her growing-up years, she had always given up something for Lent. This year
her pastor encouraged the congregation to do
something for someone during Lent. "So I took
you!" she said. What a blessing!

Pete's folks in Chicago sent a card every two
or three weeks, always wonderful little Victorian cards with Scripture written inside for my
encouragement. Aileen Ward, my eighth-grade

Sunday school teacher, often sent letters. What a blessing!

Blessings came from the Billings First Alliance Church people! We attended that church years ago when we lived in Billings. Many of those dear friends came to the Northern Rockies Cancer Center and sat there until my driver-of-the-day and I arrived. For the few minutes we had before my appointment, they visited and prayed with me. The church people gave me a scarf that had signatures and verses of encouragement written all over it, some from people I didn't know. I keep it on the shelf behind my chair in my hovel.

Another time when I got to the Cancer Center, Harold and Beulah Erickson from Bozeman, 140 miles west of Billings, were waiting for me. They had made the trip just so we could pray together. And God blessed me specially that day—that was the only day the Zapper malfunctioned and my treatment was delayed by an hour! What a blessing!

Cancer treatment facilities are as varied as the disease. Around the world, equipment to treat cancer patients is housed in a wide variety of facilities. You can be treated in a clinic, a hospital, a private doctor's office or a public or private health care building.

Some have not remodeled or updated their decor since the facility was built. Money is just not available for extras since keeping up-to-date with the medical equipment is extremely expensive. For most clinics or medical practices, the equipment and maintenance has a drastic impact on the budget. Therefore little is left for the amenities.

Many studies have revealed, however, that the setting of the treatment has a significant impact on the attitude and well-being of the patients. Many of the "charter members" of the Cancer Club that I talked with related traumatic and humiliating experiences in the olden days. Sometimes the lack of privacy and the crowded waiting areas were more taxing than the treatment itself.

I am one of the blessed ones. The Northern Rockies Cancer Center at which I was treated was designed to be "user-friendly." Every part of the building is attractive and functional. The privacy and comfort of each individual patient was a priority when they designed the building. The staff adds personal contact to ensure as pleasant an atmosphere as possible. With the ducks and the notebooks, my feeling comfortable was a given.

Then I discovered they even had a coffee machine. Pour a cup of coffee for me, give me a chair and someone to visit with and I'm happy. What a blessing!

Federal regulations and legislation by our government may change our health care system in drastic ways. We do not know the future of the rising costs of health care. My heart goes out to individuals who do not have adequate health insurance. Our family is insured through our employment. It was a blessing not to have the additional woes of huge medical bills. And there were huge costs associated with my treatment. We are still paying $50 per month to the Billings Clinic for our share of the bill that insurance did not cover.

This health crisis also made us do something we had put off year after year. We called our attorney and had a will drawn up!

Many times during treatment, my white blood count went into the basement. Then I was quarantined at home so I wouldn't catch anything. On one of these occasions, the doorbell rang. When Robert answered the door, the lawn was full of church women. He brought a chair to the front door for me. Colleen played her guitar, and for thirty minutes they sang to me! What was funny was that several neighbors immediately called our son Todd and asked if I had taken a turn for the worse? Must be an omen: When the church women come to sing on your lawn, you're a goner!

Music is one of my friend Phyllis' best gifts from God. She called during another of my housebound weeks. "I am as healthy as I know how to be," she said. "I don't think I have a germ in my body, and I haven't been around any sick people. Do you think Robert would let me come over?" Even my friends cowered under the authority of doctor-practitioner Olmstead!

"Sure, come over. I feel like I'm stranded on an iceberg. It's been a long week."

Phyllis came over, lugging her sound-machine tape-thing that enables her to sing with tapes. And for the next hour and a half she sang to me. A private concert. One that would thrill any huge audience, but the audience was just one. No, two. I'm sure God was as blessed as I was.

She handed me a cassette tape as she was leaving. "I taped this while I was singing and we were praying," she said. "Now you can play it when you need some cheering up." What a blessing!

Then there's the blessing of having friends in the same boat. A kinship that cannot be defined develops with other cancer victims. Marty Blake and Cheryl Robinson Booth were going through treatment at the same time I was. I treasure the memories. Marty died a few days before Cheryl. I imagine they already looked up my friend Jehoshaphat in heaven. I wrote about Cheryl, a Northern Cheyenne Indian, in my column.

When I found out I had cancer, I sought my friend Cheryl. I needed her. I learned from her. We often met at the Coal Bowl for milk shakes and talk.

Later my cancer responded to treatment and hers didn't. Then she needed me. So we drank more milk shakes and talked some more. A few weeks later we became "Phone Friends." Due to low white counts, we both were in isolation. She in her bed in her house. I in mine.

So we'd call—and talk and talk on the phone. We talked about cancer but we also talked about our jobs and our families. The two "phone-friends" became soul mates. No longer was the friendship based on need . . . We grew closer as we discovered all the things we had in common.

In addition to the other things, we shared the love of laughter. I would tell a funny story and we'd laugh. Then she'd add one dry comment that would be funnier than the whole story I told!

"Well, it's hard to believe we both rode horses in our time." I said to Cheryl as we were watching horses jump over fences on TV.

"Did you ever jump a fence with a horse?"

She just gave me that dry look and said, "Not on purpose!"

The most precious thing we shared was our love of Jesus. We both believed that our relationship with Jesus is based on a decision on our part—to put our trust in Him as Savior.

Many times we sang about Jesus together. As she got weaker, she had to love me a lot—because I'd sing and she'd mouth the words along with me.

The last few weeks we played "PRE-TEND"—and we took PRETEND trips.

Last Friday night she was so weak—but I told her we were going to the Bridger Mountains—up to Fairy Lake . . . I described the mountain peaks, and the trees and we took a pretend trip in a canoe on the lake . . . I told her we'd sleep under the stars.

"We'll play 'Cowboys and Indians.' " I said. She smiled a big smile and opened her eyes wide—and I knew what she was thinking. She wouldn't have any trouble being the Indian—but she was doubting I could be the Cowboy! . . .

I feel a great loss. I will miss you, Phone Friend—and I know your family is going to miss you so much more—But I KNOW you are in heaven, walking on streets of gold and flying like an eagle.

"Time Out With Lois," reprinted from the *Rosebud Press* and the *Forsyth Independent*, September 16, 1993.

The prayer partners were another blessing.

Cheryl, Pastor Mike's wife, prayed for my hair! I never lost all my hair. Toward the end of my chemo, it was plenty thin, but it never fell out completely. Les, my beautician (I have *no* talent in the hairstyle department), fixed up my wig, just in case I needed it. She used her talent every week to keep the bald places hidden. What a blessing!

Everything—my hair, the meals, the visits, the gifts—was a blessing of love I will never forget. You can tell what a sentimental creature I am because I keep the gifts and cards all around me. Robert says someday this hovel may fall off the house, it has so much stuff in it.

I know the stuff isn't what is really important: It's the thought behind it that counts! For all those "thoughts" I am humbly grateful. I pray that this book will be a testimony of not only God's miraculous working in my life, but a testimony of how much others blessed me and how you in turn can bless someone else.

As soon as I learn to cook, you can bet I am going to start taking meals to other people! Right now we just wrap a tea towel around a gift certificate to a favorite restaurant!

"You didn't say anything about appreciating our constant companionship. And we were right there all the time whispering in your ear!"

Chapter 16

No Other Foundation

For no one can lay any foundation other than the one already laid, which is Jesus Christ.
(1 Corinthians 3:11 NIV)

My husband is six feet nine inches tall. He wears size sixteen shoes. He has a standard answer when asked, "What size shoes *are* those?"

"Sixteen . . . they don't put poor foundations under quality construction, you know."

He's right. The foundation is the most important component of any building whether it is a garden shed or a high-rise office building. The same principles apply to us. How we react to a difficult time in our lives is determined by where our foundation is laid. Whether we are young or old, strong or weak, bold or shy, the most important aspect of our life is our foundation.

If the foundation in my life is built on my profession, what happens when I lose my job? Or if my foundation is built on my looks, what happens when I look in the mirror and see wrinkles or sagging skin? What if we build all our hopes and dreams on our spouse or another person and they fail to meet our expectations? Or on our athletic endeavors and abilities and an injury prevents further pursuit of sports activities?

People build their lives on many different foundations: their abilities, their spouses, performance of their children, their church affiliations or the assurance of money in the bank. Even being thin or popular or the best housekeeper in the neighborhood. Do you notice something about all of these? They can fade away or be lost or destroyed.

A foundation built on the Lord Jesus Christ is everlasting. God says in His Word, "My sheep listen to my voice; I know them, and they follow me. I give them eternal life, and they shall never perish; no one can snatch them out of my hand. My Father, who has given them to me, is greater than all; no one can snatch them out of my Father's hand" (John 10:27-29, NIV).

One of my favorite songs is a golden oldie from Sunday school days:

> The foolish man built his house upon
>   the sand . . .
> The rains came down and the floods
>   came up . . .
> And the foolish man's house fell *flat!*

> The wise man built his house upon the
> rock . . .
> The rains came down and floods came
> up . . .
> And the wise man's house stood *firm*!
>
> So build your house on the Lord Jesus
> Christ . . .
> The blessings will come down when
> the prayers go up . . .
> So build *your* house on the *Lord
> Jesus Christ!*

(That song comes from Matthew 7:24-27.)

Let's think about the similarities and the differences in human construction and God's. In construction once the foundation is laid it is done. If the workers make some mistake in the foundation, an unstable building will result.

But in life when our foundation is on Jesus Christ, we know we have a perfect beginning. We can confidently build the building of our life. We attach the bottom layer to the foundation by learning through the Holy Spirit to yield to Christ and trust Him. Our faith grows as we study the Word. Our building in Jesus Christ grows stronger as we learn to trust Him more.

In construction it is a difficult and expensive process to make significant changes in the building once the foundation is completed.

In our Christian walk as God lovingly

teaches us, He can make tremendous altera-
tions in the building of our life. He changes our
priorities as we walk with Him. And He forgives us (1 John 1:9) when we make mistakes in
placing worldly dreams and aspirations ahead
of Him.

In construction there are trends to follow.
Construction engineers learn from past meth-
ods. With new technology and bigger equipment, they design better buildings and change
our future. Yet without the trials, triumphs and
errors of those who have gone before, our
buildings would not be as strong.

Christians have a heritage too. When we
learn about godly people who have gone before us, our faith is strengthened. We gain inspiration by reading from the Bible about those
who followed Jesus. We watch others and learn
both from their victories and defeats. Without
the trials, triumphs and errors of those who
have gone before, our buildings would not be
as strong.

My foundation was well established on the
Lord Jesus Christ when cancer entered my life.
I was far from perfect, but God was in charge of
perfecting me. He was building the building.
Part of the construction of my building came
from my family heritage.

My Mom

I held my pen poised over the contest form
at Rimrock Mall. The entry blank said, "Tell

why your mom should be Queen for a Day at Rimrock Mall."

My mom has been a Montana ranch wife for over fifty years. She and Dad raised my brother and me with hard work, discipline and lots of love. My mom raised chickens and had a big garden. As I got older I realized that she didn't do this for fun; it was our groceries. She still gardens and gives my family jars of her delicious fruits and vegetables. People always think she's my sister when they meet us together because she looks so young. I tell her, "That's great for you, but I sure must be aging fast."

She tells me, "You're only as old as you feel."

She looks great when she's all dressed up for church or a speaking engagement or a dinner out with Dad. But the minute she gets home, she jumps into her Levi jeans and boots. She looks great then, too. She can cook a delicious meal when ten people pop in unexpectedly at the ranch, like they always do.

Her guest bed was occupied thirty nights in a row during hunting season by different visitors. I guess that's what motivated her to build a log guest cabin out behind the house. She peeled the logs, used the tractor and a farm-hand to lift them in place and even built the bunk beds and the outhouse (with a half moon in the door to make it authentic).

My pen was still poised midair over the entry blank.

My mom drives the hay baler and leads a Bible study. My mom can change a tire or pull a calf. She has shot deer, antelope, elk and moose. A black bear she saw is now a rug, hanging in their log home which she and Dad designed. She went on an eighty-mile trail ride in the Teton Mountains to celebrate her sixty-third birthday and loved it. When I called her a few days ago she told me she had planted 250 baby Christmas trees the day before. And she laughingly told me about being out marking the new calves when an upset mother cow went after her and Dad. She had gotten off her three-wheeler a few minutes before. Dad took a belly dive onto the haywagon and Mom scaled the pigpen fence in one leap. Thankfully no pigs were in that pen.

The entry form was still blank.

What I appreciate most about Mom is the example she set for me in being a godly wife and mother. Her faith in God through the good times and the bad has inspired my own faith.

I wiped a few tears from my eyes and crumpled up the entry blank with a smile. *Mom can't possibly be Rimrock Mall's Queen for a Day. She hasn't got time!*

My Dad

When I wrote about my mom in my newspaper column a few years ago, Dad said, "That was great, now just don't get any ideas about writing about me."

Dear Dad,

You know how difficult it has always been for me to follow your instructions. I remember how you gave me directions for chores. You told me to give two flakes of hay to the horses, feed a bucket of grain to the 4-H calves and bring in three loads of wood. You repeated it twice while I got my coat. I raced out to the barn, gave the horses two buckets of grain, fed the calves three flakes of hay and brought in one load of wood. I should have listened.

I remember when you told me not to drive the old Plymouth because it didn't have brakes. But when Mom told me to get a jug of milk from the neighbor's dairy, I jumped into the Plymouth and zoomed over the hill. Going down the first hill I remembered what you said, but it was too late. I drove like Mario Andretti over the hills and around the corners right into the neighbor's yard. I thought the only way to stop was to aim at something bigger than the car, so I headed for their barn. I knocked out three cinder blocks in the wall. I jumped out of the car and looked toward home. A cloud of dust was billowing like a hurricane down our road. You made it to my side in record time. I'm sure you thought I was killed. I should have listened.

I think you lost most of your hair when I started to date. You told me where I could go and when. You checked on my date's driving ability. You told me what time to be in and not to "park" in the yard after I got home. I didn't listen. You reminded me by blinking the yard light. I wasn't too worried about one blink, but three blinks meant my date had overextended his welcome and you would be coming out to escort him off the place!

You were very strict. I certainly got a good number of educational lessons applied to my backside when I was young. But, strict as you were, I never had a single doubt about your immense love for me.

You taught me most by example. I think I was twelve when you and Mom gave your lives to the Lord. Every night before you went to bed, you knelt by the white footstool in the living room and prayed. Every morning I saw you reading your Bible before you went out for chores. You taught me that living for the Lord was a daily walk, not just a Sunday affair. When I went to college, I knew you were praying for me. After I got married, I knew you were praying for us. Today when you are busier than ever on the ranch and working harder than ever, I know you are praying for our children, their children, me and this book. I know you told me not to write about you . . . should I have listened?

My Grandma

I learned much about relying on God and the importance of making Him the foundation of my life while writing my maternal grandmother's life story. Nancy Lennemann, my grandma, met the love of her life, Bill Adams, at a Fourth of July celebration. It was 1923.

Their wedding day was three weeks later to the day. He was twenty-three. She was four months short of eighteen. Bill was a cook. The newlyweds lived in the hotel in Clyde Park, Montana, where he worked for the first few months. Bill had "spells" with his heart now and then but their family life was good. My mom, Lorraine, was their firstborn. They moved to a small house near Bill's folks. A year later in 1924 there were some revival meetings in an empty house a couple blocks away from their home.

"We attended the meetings," Grandma said. "Together Bill and I went forward at one of the meetings and accepted Christ. This was our spiritual birth. We realized Jesus died on the cross for us. Every night we studied the Bible and Bill played a little on the guitar. We'd sing some hymns and have prayer before we went to bed."

A second baby, Alice, was born in 1926. Despite Bill's frequent spells the couple was happy. They had lots of friends and family close by. But the spells got worse. On November 30, 1926, Bill went to be with the Lord.

"This was a hard time," Grandma said. "I had just turned twenty-one. I had these two little girls. The only thing that held me up was being strong in the Lord's strength. I knew I had to take care of their future."

But the trouble wasn't over. After the funeral she felt sick. She had a high fever. When she started breaking out with a rash, the doctor said, "You have smallpox."

The grieving widow and two little girls were in their tiny house. A big yellow *Quarantined* sign was nailed to the door. Grandma's small-pox hurt and itched. She took care of her babies and dealt with the grief by talking to her Lord. They were under quarantine over Christmas and New Year's Day. Relatives brought food and milk and left it on the doorstep. Finally the quarantine was lifted. The health officer brought a type of candle that they were to burn to fumigate the house.

They had to fumigate half the house one day and the other half the next day. On the second day they had to walk outside on a freezing day, leave their clothing at the door and bathe in a tub they had prepared the day before in the now-clean kitchen.

"There wasn't much privacy taking a bath in the kitchen," Grandma said. "But I was pretty strong. God was my strength. All I could think about was taking care of these two little girls I was left with. By the next day we could open up our house. Now we were clean! We could start again. I knew I had to keep going somehow. And I knew God would take care of us."

Grandma wrote letters and called me through-out my treatment, always saying, "Hello, honey, how are you doing? I'm praying for you." At eighty-seven, she hosts a Bible study and serves others. She is a constant reminder of the necessity of a foundation built on the Lord Jesus Christ.

My Great-Aunt Ruth

My paternal grandfather's sister was the youngest of seven children born to Swedish parents. Her name was Ruth Bohleen Dickson. I just called her Aunt Ruth. She has had a tremendous impact on my life.

"We were not rich in material goods," she told me, "but rich in love and happiness over little things like an old doll dressed up new for Christmas.

"I gave my heart to Jesus," she said, "and at sixteen I sensed God calling me to full-time service for Him. I didn't know how God could use a country girl like me, but I thought maybe I could be a preacher's wife."

She went to a Christian and Missionary Alliance Bible college in 1917. She told often how God supplied the finances for this. There, God called her to be a missionary in Zamboanga, Philippines. She loved the Filipino people dearly. They called her "Mother Bohleen."

She returned to Zamboanga in 1941 after her second furlough. On a December Monday at about 6 a.m., a boy came to her door. He said the Japanese had bombed Pearl Harbor. The few missionaries gathered together.

"We read Psalm 91. We memorized it and re-peated it many times in the next three years. On January 1, 1942, we heard planes coming over. We began to sing 'God Bless America.' But then we realized they were Japanese planes. We ran to the coconut groves and hid. There were about thirty American adults and children in the group.

"The next day we packed belongings and mattresses in a truck and headed into the inte-rior. Members of the mountain Aumbouna tribe had said we could live with them. Part way there we had to abandon the truck. The tribe helped us make bamboo houses. We planted a huge garden and took turns guarding the sweet potatoes from the monkeys. I spent those hours reading the Bible."

But the Japanese found them. The missionar-ies were herded down the mountain by their captors on January 2, 1943. Aunt Ruth said she looked back and saw their camp in flames. They had only what they could carry in their arms. When they reached the Philippine shore, they were put on a boat.

"As we passed along the shore," she said, "we saw some of the boys we knew. One of them cupped his hands to his mouth. He shouted, 'Romans 8:28'! We saw them bow their heads. We knew they were praying for us."

The missionaries were kept in a large dance hall in Davao. They hung up sheets to offer a bit of privacy. "It was a filthy place," she said. "With awful outhouses and huge cockroaches. When it rained, we used shovels to clear the mud." Then she smiled, "But one thing I will never forget. There were the most beautiful sunsets!"

It was here she met Rob Dickson. He was headmaster at a boys' school. He had been transferred from another island prison. He had been ordered to dig his grave and was told it would take fifteen minutes after the bayonet pierced his body for unconsciousness to take over. Rob made a promise on that morning to serve God the rest of his life if his life was spared. Unknown to Rob, a Filipino merchant was intervening on his behalf at that time. He was sent to Davao instead of being killed.

On Christmas Day 1943, all 250 Americans at the Davao dance hall were put on a rat-infested ship. "I shall never forget the heat in that hold," Aunt Ruth said. "We got one drink of stale water daily."

They were taken to a concentration camp in Manila. There were 4,000 captives there. "It was better there," she recalled. "There was more to eat. We got one Red Cross box that had some jam and canned food. We made it last as long as we could." As a result of their starvation, the prisoners spent time recollecting and copying recipes.

"In September we heard planes coming over. American planes," Aunt Ruth said. "We thought we'd soon be out. But we spent another Christmas in prison. That Christmas Rob and I got engaged. How happy we were."

General Douglas MacArthur and the troops arrived at the end of January 1945. Rob was one of the first to be sent home because he was so ill. Ruth left the Philippines on April 1 and arrived in California by the end of the month. She and Rob were married on June 16.

They went on a camping honeymoon. She kept their grocery list for the four-day trip. I read the worn piece of paper:

4 dozen eggs	fresh vegetables
2 cans beans	2 pounds coffee
2 cans hash	1 pound ham
cakes	3 pounds beef
cheese	peanut butter
2 loaves bread	fruits

Rob remembered his promise to the Lord and served Him to the best of his ability. Rob and Ruth had seven years together before Rob died of complications from the years in prison.

Aunt Ruth went to be with the Lord on June 15, 1987. She was ninety. I received a package a few weeks later. It was her well-worn, red Bible. It is on the shelf beside me at this moment.

* * *

Can you see how my heritage could strengthen my life? And strengthen my faith in God as surely as if I had added 2" x 6"s to the foundation of my house?

Or are you thinking, *Well, fine, but I don't have a Christian background. I didn't have a great-Aunt Ruth.* That may be true. But if you attend church regularly, you can upgrade your building construction by sharing testimonies of God's mercy with others in your church. Be quick to ask how God has worked in a new acquaintance's life. I have been deeply convicted about how much time I can waste talking to a fellow believer about worldly things when that time could be much better spent talking about spiritual things. By sharing openly the victories God has given us, we can create "bricks of godly heritage" for others' buildings. That in itself can produce an atmosphere of sharing for others.

I thank God for my own heritage. I know how blessed I am. I have so many friends who are the first Christians in their families. Therefore I tell them that together we can begin building a heritage from this day forth for our own children.

We start here, right where we are. By trusting God daily. By setting godly principles to live by. Let others see us trusting in God in our weakness. By testifying through trials of how God meets your needs, you lay bricks and mortar on others' houses.

We learned, through our own family experiences, about counting our blessings each day as we walked step by step through some difficult crisis. Through the years of our life together, many times Robert and I fell before the Lord during the hard times. Other times we tried to solve the situation by ourselves—and then went to the Lord when all our attempts failed. Because of those training times, especially after Ross was in a horrible car accident, we learned *God is faithful.*

As the Bible says, "Therefore . . . "

Therefore, when the doctor said, "This tumor appears to be malignant. . . ." The rains could come down. The floods could come up. And the house on the rock could stand firm. The house had been in storms before. The structure had been tested. The building of my life had been strengthened with heavy-duty materials . . . through my heritage and the testimonies of the saints, like Mom, Dad, Grandma, Aunt Ruth . . . and Jehoshaphat.

"OK. OK. We'll pull the curtain on this play. Don't show us what the critics have to say!"

Building Application

1. Establish a journal. Begin immediately to record the victories that God has bestowed on you, your family or friends. Record it for your children and grandchildren.

"Only be careful, and watch yourselves closely so that you do not forget the things your eyes have seen or let them slip from your heart as long as you live. Teach them to your children and to their children after them" (Deuteronomy 4:9, NIV).

2. Examine with prayer and Scripture your own foundation. Working with a friend will help you be objective. You both can be blessed.

3. If there are failures and disappointments in your past, give them to God. He forgives.

1 John 1:9	Ephesians 1:6-7
2 Corinthians 5:17	Hebrews 8:12
Isaiah 55:7	Colossians 3:13

4. If you do not know Jesus Christ as your Savior and Lord, turn your life over to Him now. You have read throughout this book how many lives have been changed when they invited Him into their lives.

5. Get in a Bible study. Call pastors and interview them, visit churches until you find one with caring, compassionate people who are willing to share their lives with you. Make certain their doctrine is centered around the salvation Jesus Christ made

available to us, through grace, by His sacrifice on the cross.

Check your local Christian bookstore or write the following addresses for some correspondence Bible studies:

Stonecroft Ministries
PO Box 9609
Kansas City, Missouri 64134-0609

InterVarsity Press
Downers Grove, Illinois 60515

Chapter 17

Berachah . . .
the End Is the Beginning

*And on the fourth day they assembled them-
selves in the valley of Berachah; for there they
blessed the* LORD: *therefore the name of the
same place was called, The valley of Berachah,
unto this day.*

(2 *Chronicles* 20:26, *KJV*)

My Berachah is a log cabin in Story, Wyo-
ming. Logs, my only companions, crackle
and sparkle in the fireplace. But I am not alone.
The sweet presence of God fills this room. And
I sense the spirit of Jehoshaphat is here too.

Soon it will be four years since my treatments
for breast cancer were completed. I continue
regular three-month checkups with Dr. Lamm
and Dr. Santala and a yearly checkup with Dr.
Brown so that any reoccurrence can be de-
tected early.

But I do not live in fear. I live each day fully.
("Too fully," says Robert.) I know that my days

are in the will of my Father in heaven, just as they were before cancer was discovered in my body.

God has blessed my life beyond measure. His promises are true. "I have come that they may have life, and have it to the full" (John 10:10, NIV). I am thankful for each new day. When asked if cancer changed my life, I answer, "Yes, most assuredly."

My faith in God is more sure. I am so grateful for every blessing that at times I feel over-whelmed. My sense of God's presence is more keen. Material things do not have the same importance they used to. Don't groan; I am human. I still love to shop—I just buy less than I used to!

Robert and my family are dearer than ever before. I know how blessed I am to be married to Robert Olmstead. I still call my folks early every morning, only I no longer have to give them a cancer report. Children and grandchildren are now a priority, ahead of friends.

Am I a better person now? I don't think so. Maybe more considerate of others. Maybe a more compassionate wife, daughter and mother. Definitely not a better cook. I still can't cook! I still get moody. I still get grouchy. I still want things "my way" lots of times. And Robert says when I get in one of my Lois-on-a-mission modes, I'm still nearly impossible to live with.

I think that is why he arranged for this cabin for me to finish this writing—he didn't want to

be around me. Although I have missed him ter-
ribly, I know he's right. As usual!

Has my cancer changed our marriage? Most
decidedly so. Robert is now the spiritual *leader*
in our family. He has grown leaps and bounds
in his personal life with the Lord. We spend
more time together. We listen to each other better than before. He continually tells me to slow
down. I continually forget. But I am trying.

Robert retired this year in an early retirement
program after thirty years with Montana Power
Company. We sold our house on the lake and
bought a small place ten miles from Colstrip.
There is a big shop for Robert to play with cars.
He started his own business finding parts for
other people. He loves it. A small pond is in the
center of our ten acres. This spring I'm going to
get some more baby ducks. We cherish our
days together.

What is the downside of my cancer experience? What do I struggle with these days?

Sometimes when I least expect it, I hear those
voices:

"He-l-l-l-o-o! Here we a-r-r-e!
Coming for a rerun . . ."

But I recognize where they come from. And
again I tell myself God is in charge of my days!

My struggle is in the fact that I am still alive . . .
and Cheryl and Marty and Brad and Tommy

and Pat and Kitty and Lisa and so many other young people aren't. I cry almost every time I come out of my three-month checkups. I sit in the car and cry. Robert pats my shoulder or holds me close and understands.

"Why am I still here and they aren't?" I ask. "Why did God take them and not me?"

"I don't know, you'll just have to ask God," Robert always answers. "I still want you here."

It has been a burden for me to bear because I do not understand (and I like to understand). I can only continue to trust God that He has a plan.

Someday when I get to heaven, I will ask. One day I will go to heaven. I don't know when. I don't know if cancer will be my ticket or something else. I don't know if it will be sooner—or later. But I know I'm going. I believe God's Word. "For God so loved the world that he gave his one and only Son, that whoever believes in him shall not perish but have eternal life" (John 3:16, NIV).

When I get there, I will praise God for all eternity . . . from my valley of Berachah.

I'll be singing with Jehoshaphat (if he isn't upset with me over associating him with the breast-word).

I have a song picked out:

"To God be the glory, great things he
    hath done! . . .

> Great things he has taught us . . . through
> Jesus the Son."

Until then, for all my family and friends and cancer-patient friends, I'll be singing songs (quietly, of course) here on earth. I'll remember, as Stuart Hamblem sings in "Until Then," that "a heartache here is but a stepping stone. . . . This troubled world is not my final home."

Until then I'll sing with joy.
Can you sing along with me?

Breast cancer is not the end.
It's a new beginning.

301 Meggs Street
Copperas Cove, TX 76522

April 7, 1998

Dear Mrs. Olmstead,

I am sure you get hundreds (thousands) of letters, but I just had to tell you how important your book *Breast Cancer and Me* has been to me.

Last April I became a Christian, brought to the Lord via computer by a wonderful woman in Helena, Montana. Then in August I found out I had breast cancer. It was a true test of my newfound faith.

In September I had a mastectomy with a four-cm malignant tumor. Six lymph nodes were involved and the prognosis was very poor. I have been on chemo since October of last year and will be on it until October of this year.

My spiritual mama in Helena has been a Godsend, and I have grown in the Lord. But nobody "really" understood what I was feeling and going through. How can you have doubts and fears if you have faith in God? I heard that over and over again.

Then about a week ago my friend Helena found your book. She wasn't going to sent it to me at first, as she felt it was too "real" and might upset me. Then she said she felt the Holy Spirit tell her to get it.

I couldn't believe it. . . . It was like I had written the book. Every thought, every fear and hope you had was exactly what I had experienced and in fact am still experiencing. And the cancer talking to you. . . . That was priceless. I "hear" those cancer cells all the time, telling me that they are there—I just don't know where.

Every chapter brought tears and laughter. The bit about the wig being a dead squirrel was right on target. Nobody could understand why it upset me so. And the hot flashes were hysterical.

I guess you get the idea. I found out that I was not crazy. . . . I am normal!! And with God's help, I will make it!! And again, I thank you for taking the time to share your experiences with us.

Bless you!

Gloria Steele